Study Skills in Health Care

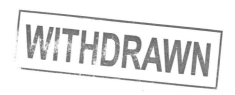

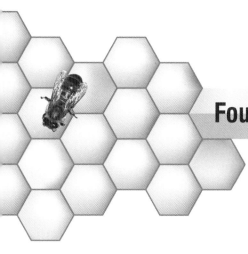

Foundations in Nursing and Health Care

Study Skills in Health Care

Jayne D. Taylor
Series Editor: Lynne Wigens

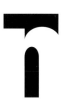

Published in 2003 by:
Nelson Thornes Ltd
Delta Place
27 Bath Road
CHELTENHAM
GL53 7TH
United Kingdom

03 04 05 06 07 / 10 9 8 7 6 5 4 3 2 1

A catalogue record for this book is available from the British Library

ISBN 0 7487 7119 0

Illustrations by Clinton Banbury
Page make-up by Florence Production Ltd, Stoodleigh, Devon

Printed in Croatia by Zrinski

Contents

Contributors

Tony Shepherd BA DMS MCILIP MCIM
Manager of Learning Resource Centre, John Kelly Technology
College, London (formerly Head of Library and Information
Services, Royal College of Nursing)

Laura Taylor RGN
Medical student, University of East Anglia, Norwich

Jayne Taylor PhD BSc (Hons) RGN RHV DipN (Lond), CertEd
MBA
Clinical Governance and Education Manager, Hertsmere PCT
(formerly Dean of the School of Health, Suffolk College)

Victoria Taylor
Law student, Christ's College, Cambridge

Stewart Taylor BSc (Hons) MIMechE
Education consultant, Edutrain 21, Suffolk

Acknowledgements

I would like to thank Stewart Taylor, Laura Taylor, Tony Shepherd and Victoria Taylor for their valuable contributions to this book. Thanks go to the 1990 RSCN students in Norwich for their help in evaluating the original works. I am grateful to Lisa Field, former editor at Harper Collins, for her support and encouragement and to Richard Holloway and Helen Broadfield for their guidance. My special thanks to Barbara Weller who, many years ago, gave me the opportunity and confidence to write.

Preface

Many students undertaking health-care programmes will have been away from a college or school environment for some time and the very nature of health-related courses means that the components of these courses are likely to be very different from anything you have studied before. Health-care practice is constantly changing and the demands on students are high in terms of the commitment needed to succeed. Whether you are just starting out in your career and embarking on a course leading to professional accreditation or you are already qualified and returning to study, this book aims to help you to cope with the academic demands of your course.

This book is designed to help you get the most out of your course. It is divided into small chapters, some of which can be read before you start and others that will be of help once your course has started. The chapters are designed so that they can be used independently.

The book was written with an appreciation of how difficult it can be to start a new course and cope with other commitments as well. Many of the hints given are founded on personal experience of trying to study and continue to do all the other things you enjoy doing. The book acknowledges that most students have families, friends, pets, hobbies and pastimes that need to be managed rather than abandoned!

Jayne Taylor
April 2003

1 Organising yourself to study

Learning outcomes

By the end of this chapter you should be able to:

- Understand the environmental factors which contribute to successful study and adapt them to your situation
- Distinguish between formative and summative assignments in your course
- Recognise Maslow's hierarchy of motivation
- Identify your own learning style.

Whether you are leaving home for the first time or you are a mature student starting your career, or you are already qualified and are about to undertake a postqualifying course, you will need to think about getting yourself organised to study. Health-related courses demand a high academic standard and usually include a practice component. For many students this will mean attending a course that extends beyond the usual term or semester structures of the university. In other words, when other 'non-health' students are heading home for the long summer vacations or having extended study time, you are likely to be spending time undertaking practice or other activities. Managing your time effectively to include studying is something that requires careful thought if you are to be successful in gaining the qualification you require.

You may be quite used to organising your study time if you have fairly recently left school or have undertaken an educational course. However, your health-care course may be combined with your first time away from home and you need to balance additional demands on your time, such as shopping for food, cooking, washing and ironing as well as all the more pleasant demands, such as parties, the cinema, the pub, etc. You will need to set aside sufficient time for study if you are to fulfil the requirements of your course successfully. It is all too easy to fill your time up with various activities and lose sight of what you are actually hoping to achieve.

It may have been a long time since you have had to think about organising your time to include studying as well as all the other activities you are involved with. We tend to lead full lives involving social, domestic, occupational and family-related activities. Additional time for studying doesn't necessarily mean giving up some or all of your other commitments but it will mean readjusting your busy schedule so that studying is not neglected. If you are a mature student, becoming a health-care practitioner may have been a long-term personal ambition and the commitment to studying has been made after careful consideration. It is both frustrating and disappointing if your ambitions cannot be realised because you have not fully thought through the implications of undertaking an academic course.

> ## Over to you
>
> Using a diary and working in hour time-slots, map out your 'typical week' when you are not studying. Be honest about how much time you spend watching television, etc. Identify with a highlighter pen the times when you are most likely to be able to undertake individual study. What will you need to alter in your 'typical week' to make time for your health-care studies?

This chapter offers some hints about how you can organise yourself to maximise your potential for studying. Ultimately, though, we are all individuals and you will have to make your own decisions according to space, existing commitments and the amount of studying required by the course you are following. It is, however, worth thinking about your circumstances and how best to organise yourself at an early stage during the course, or ideally before it begins, rather than waiting until you have work to do and deadlines to meet. While most higher education institutes will give you some time to settle in to your new environment, it is likely to be only a few days, as most courses require you to prepare for lectures, **seminars** or assignments shortly after the commencement of the course.

There are several areas that need to be considered when thinking about getting yourself organised and these are summarised in Figure 1.1.

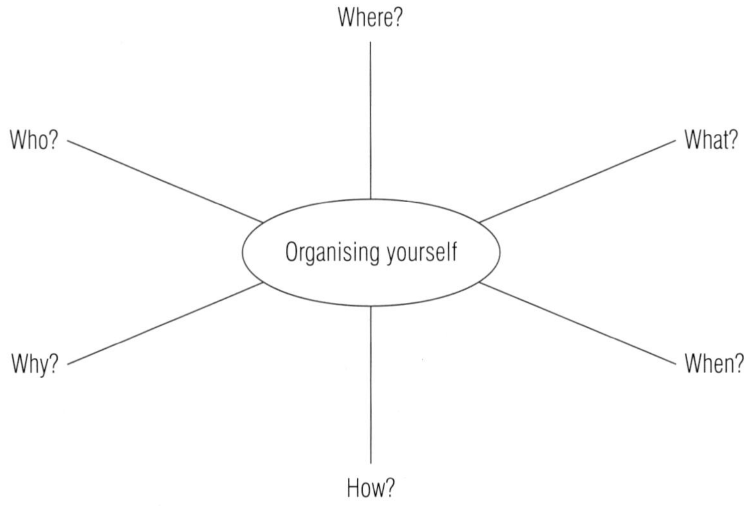

Keywords

Seminar
A class, organised by a student or tutor, that promotes discussion about a particular topic

Figure 1.1 *Areas to be considered when organising yourself to study*

Where?

You will need *somewhere* to study! The venue will depend on your own circumstances, the type of study and the time you have available. The following section highlights some important considerations.

Comfort

I have often sat down with the good intention of studying for a set period of time and then wasted half of it because I haven't been comfortable. It is very easy to make excuses for *not* studying because you need a drink or you are hungry or you are just *not* settled enough to get down to some really useful brain activity.

It is important that the environment is comfortable and you are able to study in comfort. Most residences provide basic single accommodation, which will include a desk and chair. If you live at home it is worth trying different chairs to see which is the most comfortable – the most unlikely looking chair may be the one that best suits your needs.

Wherever you live, you should think about the environmental temperature. Try not to sit in a draught or too near a radiator. (One is likely to give you a stiff neck, the other will send you to sleep!) It is worth making sure you have additional layers of clothing to put on or take off as again it is easy to use being too hot or too cold as an excuse to stop working. Lighting should also be considered and it is worth investing in a study lamp if you don't already have one. If you are moving into residence it is worth investing in an extension lead or two so that you can move furniture around to make the best use of the light and heat in your accommodation. Get these before you go as you will find that local stores tend to get depleted of such items very quickly at the start of the academic year.

It is important that you are able to keep yourself supplied with food and drink without having to leave your study environment every time you want a cup of coffee.

Company

Most student accommodation is designed so that each student has an individual room with use of communal cooking, bathing, laundry and recreational facilities. It should, therefore, be possible for you to study on your own if you want to. If your neighbours are persistently noisy, try to negotiate some rules with the people around you.

If you live at home it may be more difficult for you to be on your own, either because there is not the space or because you prefer to study while your family and friends are present so that you do not totally isolate yourself. It depends how easily distracted you are, but earplugs are the answer for some people (a handy item if you have noisy neighbours in residence). From personal experience of studying at home with young children, I have found that they are less likely to disturb me if I am with them. A closed study or dining room door seems to attract a constant stream of small visitors! If you are settling down to study with children make sure that they are also supplied with refreshments otherwise you can guarantee that someone will want a drink within minutes!

Disturbance

If you live in residence or at home there may be times when you have to say 'Please do not disturb'. A sign on the door in residence will often make friends think twice, especially if you give a time when you will be finished. Leave a pencil and paper for messages.

If you live at home, and particularly if you have children, it can be extremely difficult to arrange for undisturbed time unless you are

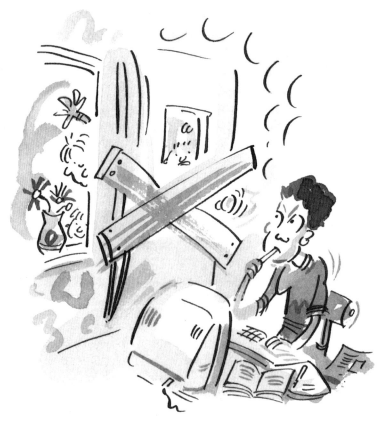

Choose a place to study that is appropriate to your situation and needs

able to work late in the evening or early in the morning. Alternatively, you can ask a trusted adult to take children off your hands for a few hours or get together with other students who are in the same position as you and childmind for each other.

It is also useful to remember that universities will have a library, which should have a silent area where you can study in peace. It is worth considering using this facility, especially if you need to refer to literature in order to complete your studying or if you find you are easily distracted by your environment.

Space

When you are in the full throes of studying it is useful to have somewhere to leave books open and to have journals and other material at hand. If you don't want a helpful friend to tidy them up for you then put a note on the work to say so. Likewise if you are studying in the library and go for a break, put a notice on your table to stop people disturbing your carefully sought references.

Key points / ***Top tips***

Studying conditions
- Be comfortable before starting to study. Don't be too hot, cold, hungry or thirsty and ensure you have adequate light to study by.
- Try and ensure you have somewhere to study in private, appropriate to your situation and lifestyle.
- Don't be afraid to say to friends and family that you don't want to be disturbed while you study. It helps to give an end time to your study session after which you will be available.

Who?

Whether you study on your own, in pairs or in a group will vary according to the work you are doing. If you work on your own, make sure you have thought through the aspects of the environment mentioned above.

If you have to work in a group certain potential problems can occur that are worth considering. Firstly, decide on the most suitable venue and who is going to find what information. It is very frustrating to meet in someone's house only to find that no-one has brought a vital piece of reference material. Then negotiate who is going to produce what and by when. Once these targets are set they should be seen as a contract. This should ensure that everyone pulls their weight. It is very easy to get distracted and frustrated if targets are not met but at least, if they have been set and agreed, all the members of the team will know who is and who is not producing the work. A good tip to remember is that courses are not a competition to see who can produce the best work in the fastest time. A hidden element of group work is to encourage you to work as a team – which is designed to equip you for working in health-care settings later on. In practice no-one can work alone so treat group work as a means of equipping yourself to deal with all sorts of people in the future. It is useful, too, if you stop to reflect on your own behaviour within group work and ask your peers to evaluate your performance. Were there things you did that upset people? Are there things that you said that irritated others? What strengths did you have in the group that you might build on for the future?

If you do find you are getting frustrated with each other, it is better to discuss the situation openly rather than having a quiet moan – that doesn't help anyone! Be honest and constructively critical with each other.

When you have completed your respective parts of an assignment, it is important to sit down and 'edit' your joint work, ensuring that the presentation and writing styles are similar and that you have not duplicated any information. Many group efforts have lost valuable marks because they have a 'thrown together' look, even though individuals have worked hard.

When considering 'Who' it is worth mentioning the staff of the university who are there to help and support you. Most universities will allocate you a personal tutor and some will have tutor groups. Your personal tutor is there to guide you through your experience on the programme and may or may not be from the discipline that you are studying. Tutors are vital people who can help you if you get into difficulty – but they will only know you are having problems if you actually tell them. They can guide you as to what processes you must follow if you miss a class or are going to have trouble meeting an assessment deadline.

Usually, your personal tutor will be a member of the lecturing staff. Lecturers, apart from lecturing and acting as personal tutors, also have other responsibilities to fulfil, such as undertaking research, writing books and so on. Universities tend to be very different from school, where teachers are likely to be around most of the time and teach for the majority of the week. If you need to see a lecturer or your personal tutor you may need to leave a message to arrange a mutually convenient time. Don't rely on them being available in their offices at your beck and call – because they won't be. They also tend to take on much more of a facilitative role, rather than providing you with all the facts that you need to get through the course, as school teachers do. You will find that you are taught for a lot less time than you were at school and are expected to spend a lot more time studying on your own or in a group.

Key points **Top tips**

Working with other people
- When working in groups, decide who is going to complete what aspect of the study and by when.
- For work completed by a group, ensure you also edit it as a group to ensure consistency of style and to avoid duplications.
- Don't forget to consult with your tutor if you are having difficulty with an aspect of study. But make sure you arrange an appointment – don't just turn up expecting them to be there!

What?

Most courses are divided into parts called units or modules and each part will usually be assessed both formatively and summatively.

☞ Keywords

Formative work
Provides feedback on your progress and development and doesn't contribute to the overall assessment of your course (QAA 2000)

Formative assessment

Formative work has several functions:
- It aims to maximise learning.
- It should build on your strengths and should enable both you and the lecturer to identify weaknesses and identify individual learning needs.
- It should encourage students to reflect on their learning and identify strategies for improvement.

Formative work has to be completed and will still be assessed even although it does not contribute to your overall course marks. Formative work is vitally important in the process of the course and, because you do not risk failing the course as a result of formative work, it also allows you to use your flair and initiative. It should help you and your lecturer identify areas where you need additional help.

☞ Keywords

Summative work
Provides a measure of performance achievement or failure in relation to learning outcomes for a particular course or part of a course (QAA 2000)

Summative assessment

There will be various assessments throughout the course, which are classed as **summative work**.

Summative assessment must be passed if you are to complete the course successfully. The Quality Assurance Agency Code of Practice requires that universities and colleges have clearly identified criteria relating to the conduct, content and standard of assessments (QAA 2000). You will usually be required to complete one part of the course successfully before you can progress to subsequent parts.

Each institution has guidelines about the number of times you can attempt summative work and it is worth finding this out before you undertake assignments or sit examinations. Depending on the institution's ruling, you will usually be given the opportunity to do remedial work with tutorial support if you fail a summative assessment. It is better, however, to seek help before assignment deadlines or before sitting an examination if you feel you are having difficulties. Many universities have a policy about allowing extensions in the case of what are often called 'mitigating circumstances' (things such as illness, which may affect your ability to submit work on time), so you must let an appropriate person know if you are having problems. Some universities will automatically deduct marks if you submit work late and may refer or fail work altogether if you miss deadlines without due cause.

Over to you

Write down your personal strategy for completing the summative and formative work for the first term/semester of the course (use this to keep yourself on track during the course).

Identify what you think might be the main things that will stop you succeeding – then try and identify strategies for overcoming each of the points you identify.

Key points | **Top tips**

Managing difficulty with summative work

- Find out your institution's guidelines as to how often you can sit examinations and other summative assignments if you fail them.
- Don't forget to seek help from your tutor *before you submit the work* if you are having difficulty with an assignment.
- If you feel you have mitigating circumstances that prevent you from submitting work on time, tell your tutor.

When?

When you should study very much depends on the aspects of getting organised already mentioned. If you are working with colleagues, you will need to negotiate to suit all concerned. However, individual study time can be worked in to suit your other commitments and you should aim to study when you know you are at your best. For example, some people find it impossible to work late at night and prefer to get up early and study then.

It is obviously important that you eat sensibly and get adequate rest, and relaxation and leisure time should also be worked out. Abraham Maslow (1954) proposed an interesting theory that looked at motivation and is particularly applicable here. This is shown in Figure 1.2. He identified that humans have a hierarchy of needs which dominate our motives. If basic needs such as hunger and thirst are not satisfied then higher motives will not seem significant. The needs at one level must be at least partially satisfied before those at the next level become important. In practical terms, if basic needs of hunger and thirst are not satisfied, you may find it difficult to motivate yourself to pursue your intellectual interests.

If you already lead a busy life you may find that, with the additional studying, you will have to spend less time in pursuit of hobbies. Don't be tempted to give up such things altogether – hobbies, especially those involving exercise, help you to relax and

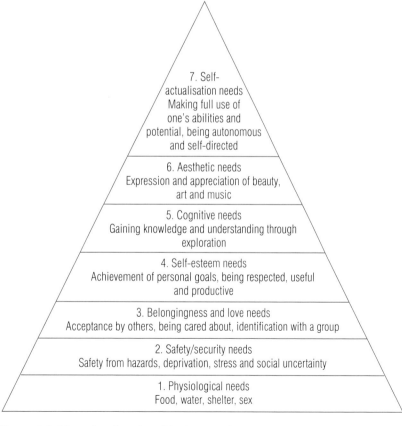

Figure 1.2 *Hierarchy of motives (Maslow 1954)*

reduce stress. As I know from personal experience, if you study late in the evenings it's a good idea to have a break and watch television, listen to some music or take a relaxing bath before you try to go to sleep.

The amount of time you spend studying will vary as the course goes on. The time you can usefully spend studying depends on you. You will need to get to know how long you can work without a break before you lose concentration. Some students find they work best if they have frequent breaks while others find that they can work for longer periods. As you get more used to studying you should be able to build up your concentration time. You may also find that, if you have several areas that you need to study, it is better to spend short periods of time on each activity so that you introduce some variety into your studying. If there is something you really don't want to do, try to spend a limited period of time doing it and reward yourself by doing something you find more interesting.

Key points **Top tips**

When to study
- Try and identify your study style. Do you work better earlier or later in the day? For long periods at a time or for more frequent, but shorter bursts? Finding this out will make your studying more effective.
- Make sure your basic needs such as hunger and thirst are dealt with before you try to settle down to study.
- If you exercise regularly, try not to give this up just because you now have to fit in some study time too.
- If you study late in the evenings, make an effort to relax before trying to go to sleep.

How?

Getting yourself organised and into the swing of things requires individual planning and will vary according to the demands of your course and your other commitments. However, a few suggestions are offered below. These suggestions are made from personal experience of spending 23 of the last 27 years studying various courses!

- Have a notebook in which to write down assignments, seminars, tutorials, etc. Ensure that you record the title, guidelines for submission, suggested word limit and date of submission as well as whom you should go to if you experience any difficulties with the work.

- Draw up a timetable for your activities each week. Start by putting in priority events (e.g. weddings, school plays, etc.) and then mark in study time. From personal experience, it always takes longer to complete assignments than you think, so add a third extra time on top of your estimated time required for study.

- Set yourself targets for completion of work. If you have several pieces of work to complete over a period of time, you may find it useful to set short- and long-term targets. Work towards short-term targets but gather reference material and other resources for your longer term targets.

- If you fail to meet your own deadlines then decide what you are going to give up in order to complete the work.

- When you complete work, reward yourself (no suggestions as to how!).

- Keep a box with index cards or set up a file on your word processor where you write down references and other useful information. It will save you time later on.

- Make sure all the important people in your life are informed of your study schedule – it saves you and them becoming frustrated, irritated and hungry!

Knowing what to do in order to organise yourself to study is only a part of the story, however. Knowing what sort of learner you are is also important and not something we tend to consider. If you think about it, you will realise that others seem to enjoy different forms of learning from you. What you might consider an easy process they might consider difficult and *vice versa*. Of course, on any course it is impossible for teachers to please all of the people all of the time, but if you are at least aware of what type of learner you are it may help.

Learning styles have been described by a number of psychologists dating back to the start of the 20th century and various methods of defining learning styles have been developed. One you may come across is Kolb's learning style inventory (Kolb 1976, Kolb and Wolfe 1981). Kolb and colleagues describe four types of people according to their learning styles. These are divergers, assimilators, convergers and accommodators. Figure 1.3 outlines some of the attributes of the four types. It is well worth using Kolb's inventory to discover for yourself where you fit in. This exercise can be more wholly completed in another book in the Foundations in Nursing and Health Care series, *Beginning Reflective Practice* by Melanie Jasper.

If nothing else, it is useful to be able to reflect on why you do or don't find particular types of learning easy. Remember, no one

Diverger	Accommodator
• Will take in information in a concrete manner and process it reflectively. • Will listen with an open mind. • Will be sensitive to other's feelings and values	• Will take in information in a concrete manner and process it actively. • Will seek and exploit opportunities. • Will lead and influence others. • Will be 'hands on' and can 'deal' with people.
Assimilator	Converger
• Will start with an idea and develop it reflectively. • Will take an analytical approach to processing information. • Will test theories and ideas.	• Will start with an idea and develop it actively. • Will create new ways of doing things. • Will experiment with new ideas. • Will set goals and make decisions.

Figure 1.3 *Different learning styles*

Reflective activity

Using Figure 1.3, try and identify what type of learner you are. Do your current learning activities really reflect your style? What do you think you will need to change in order that they do?

learning style is better than another – it is just a way of recognising that we are different and learn in different ways.

Why?

Finally, we come to the why . . . .

Students do survive courses by muddling along, leaving work until the last minute, burning the midnight oil, searching through the library to find elusive references at the eleventh hour and getting little sleep and relaxation. However, being a student is not something you should merely survive. Although you want the qualification at the end of the course, the process by which it is gained is as important as the actual product. Getting organised should be something you do for you, your friends and family. It is about getting the best out of yourself. It is about enjoying the course, meeting new people and meeting new challenges.

Rapid recap

Check your progress so far by working through each of the following questions.

1. Make of list of things you should do to make sure you are comfortable in your study environment.
2. Identify three things that you should consider when working in a group with other students.
3. Identify the seven sections of Maslow's hierarchy of motivation.
4. What is the difference between formative and summative assessment?

If you have difficulty with more than one of the questions, read through the section again to refresh your understanding before moving on.

References

Kolb, D. (1976) *Learning Style Inventory: Technical manual*. McBer & Co., Boston, MA.

Kolb, D. and Wolfe, D. (1981) *Professional Education and Career Development: A cross sectional study of adaptive competencies in experiential learning*. Department of Organizational Behavior, Case Western Reserve University, Cleveland, OH.

Maslow, A. (1954) *Motivation and Personality*. Harper & Row, New York.

QAA (2000) *Code of Practice for the Assessment of Academic Quality and Standards in Higher Education: Assessment of students*. Quality Assurance Agency, Gloucester.

2

Managing your finances

Learning outcomes

By the end of this chapter you should be able to:

- Understand eligibility for receiving student grants
- Understand the procedure for applying for a loan
- Find out if you are exempt from paying tax on your earnings

Unless you have either extremely generous relatives or an offshore bank account, money is likely to be of great importance to you while studying in higher education. The bottom line is that you won't have much of it. However there are several ways to save those precious pennies and ensure that you have enough of them to go to the pub occasionally.

Student loans

To achieve that elusive Midas touch it is important to get your finances sorted before heading off in pursuit of academia. A student loan is a good place to start. Most students can apply and will receive at least 75% of the maximum amount (a tidy sum indeed). If your (or your parents') income falls below a certain amount, you may even be eligible to have your tuition fees paid by the local education authority [LEA] but the most any home students will have to pay is one-third of tuition fees. Recent reforms to the university fee system have not been greeted enthusiastically but childcare, book and travel grants exist to ensure that no potential students are excluded from higher education because of financial problems. In other words, money is available from the government and local education authorities and they will part with it eventually (after you have filled out hundreds of forms).

Before you receive any student loan you have to be assessed by the LEA. They will request information on your course and its duration as well as information on your (or your parents') income. Once you have answered all their questions they will assess your claim and decide what percentage of tuition fees you must pay and how much of the student loan you are eligible for. Then the student loan company sends you some more forms and you decide how much (if any) of the loan you want to receive. You may decide that the loan is worth taking out because of the extremely low rate of interest charged on it. The money does need to be paid back at some

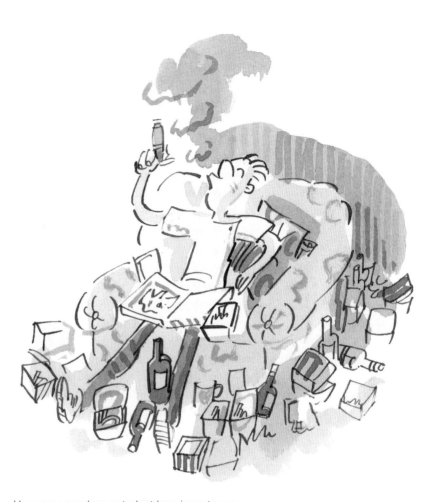

How you spend your student loan is up to you

point but not until your income rises above a certain level and even then the repayments are small.

If you do take out a student loan then you need to find it a good home (under your mattress is not a good idea!). A student bank account has various advantages and disadvantages. The main advantages are that you may get an interest-free overdraft and a credit card. The main disadvantages are that you may get an interest-free overdraft and a credit card! It is very easy to spend money that you do not really have and, as many banks charge interest of upwards of 20%, it is a good idea to keep a tight rein over your finances, however boring and un-student-like that may seem.

High street banks will try to entice you with promises of free money, CD players, popcorn makers and other such wondrous gifts. Remember, however, that nothing is really free and banks love students, who will one day earn lots of money *and* have a mortgage *and* a loan on a new car. To the bank you are merely potential earning power (see the pound signs in the bank manager's eyes when you declare you want to open an account!) and as such they will try to sell you anything and everything.

Among the best free gifts to go for are railcards, which are very useful and will allow you to drop your washing off at home at a reduced rate. They entitle you to one-third off most train journeys.

Health-care students in receipt of a bursary

○━╥ Keywords

Bursary
A grant or payment awarded to a student

Some health-care students will be eligible for a means-tested or non-means-tested **bursary**. If this applies to you, you will not be entitled to a student loan. Instead, you will receive a government-funded sum of money to support your studies. This is only fair, as you will probably have to stay on at university long after most other students have retreated home to summer jobs and home cooking.

Means-tested bursaries are assessed on income and you may or may not be eligible. You may not, however, have to pay fees. Students in receipt of a full bursary and fees-only bursary students may access the NHS Hardship Grants Scheme. Non-means-tested bursaries mean that, even if you have won the lottery and have put your winnings in the bank, you will still be entitled to the money. There are a number of rates:

- A standard rate for non-mature students without dependants living outside London
- A rate for mature students without dependants living outside London
- A rate for non-mature students without dependants living in London
- A rate for mature students without dependants living in London.

As you can probably deduce from the above if you have dependants you get more money.

You may also be entitled, as a health-care student, to receive money for travel to placements and you should definitely not have to pay for those flattering uniforms (the government got very upset when some universities tried this). Some universities will even give you a lap-top!

Tax

Tax is worth considering too. If you are a student and you don't plan to undertake part-time work during your studies to supplement your grant/bursary, you can fill in a tax exemption form to ensure that the

Inland Revenue does not accidentally remove your precious pennies. If you do work, then you need to find out if you earn enough money to have to pay tax on your earnings. Talk to your employer and your bank and they will be able to steer you through the complicated world of taxation and make sure that you don't wake up to any letters from the Inland Revenue demanding money. Students are also exempt from paying council tax.

One non-essential item that the majority of people own but that must be paid for is a television. Contrary to popular belief, even if you live in a hall of residence you must have your own television licence and, if you get caught without one, expect a four-figure fine and even a court appearance.

Owning a television, a computer or a stereo system will also make you a tempting target for thieves, so insurance is also a good idea. General cover will leave you well protected but if you own an expensive mobile, bicycle or computer it could be worth arranging extra cover. Check your home contents insurance before you arrange insurance as you might already be covered, and remember to read the small print – having to pay an excess of £50 on your mobile phone is all very well providing your mobile is actually worth more than that!

Key points **Top tips**

What you are entitled to
- Check if you are eligible to receive funding for travel expenses to placements and uniforms
- Check with your employer and/or bank whether you earn enough to have to pay tax
- Don't forget to insure your valuables: television, stereos, CDs etc.

Most students enjoy socialising, eating, drinking, shopping and a number of other extracurricular activities (none of which have any educational value at all). If you find yourself in a similar position it may be worth joining the National Union of Students (NUS). This involves very little effort and you will be rewarded with a plastic card proudly bearing your name, a dodgy photograph and the fact that you are a student (or a least pretending to be one). This small piece of plastic is your direct route to discounts on shopping, eating and drinking and you may find that it can save you quite a lot of money. It can even get you discounts on books and other educational resources. Using your NUS card will soon become second nature to you (if only they gave you frequent flyer miles) and it is worth using.

Managing your money

On a more serious note, it is very easy when you have money to get in the habit of spending it and it is amazing how many good bargains there are around. It is also easy *not* to open those bank statements when they arrive and to ignore demands from people you have borrowed money from. If and when you do decide to open your bank statements, check them carefully and learn how to read them. Don't be like the student who kept telling her father that she had loads of money – not realising that her accumulating wealth was actually an accumulating debt. 'OD' actually means overdrawn, not just overdose.

Key points | **Top tips**

Managing your money
- Make a list of essential purchases and put them in order of priority according to when you will need to buy them.
- Remember, you can actually ask for things such as books and toiletries for Christmas and birthdays.

It is obviously really important to keep tabs on what is being spent – boring though it might seem. However, most students find this a difficult skill to master. Your bank statement is a good indicator of how to lay out a simple balance sheet and, if you can, it's a good idea to create a spreadsheet on your computer. You simply need to enter what you have coming in and what you have spent and hopefully make sure the former exceeds the latter (somehow it never does – one of life's great mysteries). Remember transactions like standing orders – they will be deducted at set times in the month until you instruct your bank not to continue paying them (unless they are for purchases with a fixed repayment period).

If you have problems

Unfortunately it is true that some students do suffer real hardship. Tuition fees remain unpaid and rent arrears soon add up. Credit cards are past their limits and despair has set in. Do not panic. Universities have teams dedicated to problems such as these, usually known as Student Support Units. Welfare advisors will be happy to talk through your problems and may be able to help you make a claim through the Hardship fund. Money is available to those who really need it and it is not worth dropping out of your course because

> ## Over to you
>
> - Identify any standing orders and other automatic debits from your bank account
> - Identify any credits to your account
> - Check the appropriate booklet (see Further Reading) and make sure you are claiming everything you are entitled to
> - Set up a simple balance sheet, identifying how much you will have to spend on a monthly basis

of financial difficulties. These can be resolved – all you have to do is ask for help.

In conclusion, money is often the biggest worry for students. However, university is supposed to be fun and you must not let financial worries plague the next 3–5 years of your life. Try to achieve a balance. You do not need to go out every night but you do need to go out at least once a week. You will probably find yourself in the same position as most other students at university – overworked and underpaid – but do not let this ruin your time there. The whole point of higher education is that it will allow you to get a good job in the future. You want to be able to look back on your student years and laugh, incredulous that you actually survived.

Rapid recap

Check your progress so far by working through each of the following questions.

1. What are the grants available to ensure that no student is excluded from higher education?
2. What are the four different rates for the NHS Bursary Scheme?
3. What does NUS stand for?

If you have difficulty with any of the questions, read through the section again to refresh your understanding before moving on.

Further reading

Department for Education and Skills (2002) *Financial Support for Higher Education Students*. DES, London.

Department of Health (2000) *Financial Help for Health Care Students*, 5th edn. DoH, London.

Information and library skills

The 'information explosion' continues apace. In the last few years, there is no doubt that many thousands of books, articles, pamphlets, theses and information databases have been produced for the benefit of health-care students. The ability to find, understand and put into practice the information located in these sources is increasingly appreciated by professionals as part of their personal development. Knowing how to search effectively for the sources of ideas, arguments and information, and then decide if they are relevant or not, places the student in a strong position (Marland 1991). With the growth in the concept of 'continuing education', we are all students now and the requirement to maintain professional competence is often enshrined in employment contracts and continuing professional registration. Improved access to information means that some patients are becoming better informed, thus leading to their expectation that health-care professionals should continue their professional development.

The approach taken here is that developing information and library skills is appropriate for all methods of learning. This includes e-learning, as well as learning on full-time taught courses and learning in order to update existing knowledge. This chapter will provide guidance to enable you to make effective use of the range of sources of information available.

Planning an information search

The first stage in any information search is to plan in a structured way so as to make the best use of your time. Think carefully about your precise subject or topic and note down the main keywords or terms covering it. As your search process develops you will need to add new keywords and **synonyms** to your list. This is a normal part of the process and will enable you to sharpen your thinking about the subject in hand. It is often helpful to undertake some background reading so as to find keywords and synonyms – especially

◯━╥ Keywords
....

Synonym
A word with the same meaning as another

if the topic is new to you. It may be helpful to gain a quick overview of the subject by browsing through some relevant websites or textbooks, especially if it is a new topic subject to you.

Key points **Top tips**

Before starting your search, consider:

- Are you searching for an in-depth range of detail or for an outline search, or for some 'in between' level?
- What period of time are you going to cover?
- Which geographic area are you going to include? Obviously, a worldwide search will be more demanding.
- Will you include data from statistical records, original research, websites or newspaper files, etc.?
- How much time realistically will you have available for your search? Your research will be reduced if your time is limited.

Providers of information

The following list provides only an indication of providers in the UK and demonstrates the range of organisations that produce information in the public domain. Most of these institutions provide a library and information service (LIS) as well as publishing information of their own.

- **Government departments**. The UK government's Internet gateway is www.gov.uk. This means that all UK government website addresses will end with '.gov.uk'.
- **Department of Health**: www.doh.gov.uk.
- **The NHS** has the Internet gateway www.nhs.uk. This site provides links to the NHS across England, Scotland, Wales and Northern Ireland. There are Regional Health Service LIS networks and your local LIS should have full details.
- **Universities and Colleges**. Details can be found via your Internet search engine (e.g. Altavista or Yahoo), or from reference directories available in your LIS. As an example of one academic website, Queens University Belfast is at www.qub.ac.uk. Websites for universities give access to their LIS facilities and databases.
- **Professional bodies and unions**. Again, details can be obtained by searching using search engines, directories or links supplied by other information providers. For instance, the website

for the Royal College of Midwives (RCM) Information Centre offers links to other sources, e.g. to relevant reports on midwifery topics. The RCM is at www.rcm.org.uk. On this site, 'the library and archives' pages are found via a link on the 'information centre' page. The Royal College of Nursing (RCN) is at www.rcn.org.uk. The Community Practitioners and Health Visitors Association is at: www.amicus-cphva.org.

- **Public libraries**. As a resident you have the right to use your local public library, where you should find a wide range of resources. You can also use the interlibrary loan network available via this local library, but again you must plan ahead. Public libraries usually have a website as part of the local authorities service.

- **Other educational providers and charities** may have relevant information, e.g. Learn Direct: www.learndirect.co.uk. An example of a charity website is Oxfam's at www.oxfam.org.uk.

- **Research organisations and 'think tanks'** publish a range of material and normally have useful websites as part of their information provision, e.g. the Kings Fund is at www.kingsfund.org.uk.

- **International and non-UK information providers** may be useful, particularly if you are undertaking a large-scale or comparative study. You can search for websites in the same way as noted above, e.g. the World Health Organization is at www.who.int.

Before visiting any LIS for the first time, it is essential to check on the accessibility of the services available. Some membership organisations may charge for visitor's tickets.

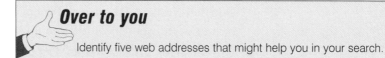

Over to you

Identify five web addresses that might help you in your search.

The range of information sources available

It is important to think about the variety of information sources available. Now is the chance to extend your skills so that you become efficient in using a range of resources. Research skills are required to maintain your professional awareness and may become

Top tips

When visiting a Library Information Service, check:
- Opening hours
- Range of resources held
- Databases available
- Librarian or specialist help available
- Which journals are available
- Obtaining articles not in stock
- Access to inter-library loans
- Computer and photocopying access

part of your general 'life skills'. You will be able to access some resources via any domestic computer with a modem through access to the Internet. Using LIS facilities normally provides access to a greater range, with the advantage of help from the library and information staff on site. Sources include the following:

Print sources

These include books, journals, research and theses materials and pamphlets.

Full text databases

These include all the above. They are normally paid for on subscription or access comes as part of membership of, for instance, the RCN. Some CD-ROMs are produced that give access to full text information as well as to bibliographical data. Look at the 'subject search' option and see if you can use the 'advanced search' option.

Audiovisual sources

These include videos, audio cassettes, CDs, video cassettes, DVDs, coloured slides and 'media packages'. Access to live and recorded video conferencing facilities, as well as audio and telephone conferences, are all part of the exchange of information. Text and picture messaging via your mobile phone should also be considered as providing access to information sources.

Bibliographical sources

These provide details of literature and are essential in the transfer of information. They include various types of database.

Bibliographic databases

Most LISs provide a database 'catalogue' of their literature and other resources on their computer system. In addition, you should look at *BNI* (the British Nursing Index) and *CINAHL* (the Cumulative Index to Nursing and Allied Health Literature) for a wide range of nursing and related literature.

For all databases, look at the 'About' introductory screens as well as at any 'guides' produced by the LIS about these key sources. They usually offer useful information about the types of service the site offers. It is also very useful to try out any 'tutorial' unit provided on the database, as well as the 'Help' option, if you have a problem. These are available online and also in CD-ROM format. You can search using a variety of approaches such as 'keyword', 'author', title or 'series'.

It is recommended that you attend any training sessions provided by your college or department on finding information or using databases.

Card catalogues

Some services still use a card catalogue for some or all of their resources. These probably include details under 'subject' ('classified'), 'authors', and 'titles' sections, as well as a 'subject index'. Use any guidance facilities provided to make the best use of these.

Printed bibliographies and abstracts

These have the same purpose as card catalogues and work in a similar way. Your local LIS will inform you of their holdings when requested. Abstracts provide a summary of the contents of documents and they appear also in full-text journals on the Internet, as in the case of the *Journal of Advanced Nursing* at www.journalofadvancednursing.com.

Other information sources

As a health-care practitioner today, you will have to be an active learner so as to retain your professional credibility, to say nothing of retaining your registration! General awareness and good practice will require some knowledge of information resources and you need to be aware that some sources are still only available in print format.

Other useful resources include the following. Examples of titles are provided by way of demonstration only.

- **Directories and yearbooks**, including *Hospital and Health Services Yearbook* (only in print format) and *Social Services Yearbook* (available on CD-ROM)

> ### Over to you
> Using an internet search engine (e.g. Google, Yahoo) find the websites for BNI and CINAHL. What types of information do they offer?

- **Reports**, including the *Nursing and Midwifery Council Annual Report, Designed to Care: Renewing the NHS in Scotland*
- **Statistics**, including data from the Office for National Statistics – *Annual Abstract of Statistics* is one example
- **Guides to periodicals**, including *Ulrich's International Periodical Director, Willings Press Guide* (especially for the UK)

Develop a search strategy

As you look at the information sources, you should refer back to your list of keywords and synonyms, which you will modify as you progress. You will need to convert your list of keywords so that they fit in with those used in the various sources. Terminology may vary in non-UK sources.

> ### Over to you
> Compare the thesaurus used in the BNI with the subject headings used in CINAHL. What are the main differences?

As you note relevant and 'possibly relevant' information, you must keep a note of your references, for use with your essay, thesis or whatever document you are producing. You will probably find it helpful to use a computer as you do this. If you don't have access to a computer, try using a set of index cards, one per reference. You will need to rearrange your references eventually into your final reference list and/or bibliography, depending upon what recording mechanism you're using.

With each reference, in a note field on your computer or on the back of your cards, note the sources where you found your reference in case you need to double-check the details later. If you are able to use a database package on your computer, such as Microsoft Access®, you could make a 'reference record' template.

Top tips

When planning your search:
- Decide upon the boundaries of the information required e.g. the range, depth, geographical spread and time available for you to carry out the work.
- Think about the providers of information and if their resources are appropriate for your needs.
- Review the range and type of sources available and decide which may be relevant.

○━┱ *Keywords*

Gateway
A website dedicated to a specific subject area and intended to provide access to a number of other websites on the topic

The use of gateways on the Internet

Gateways are valuable in that they provide a ready-made entry point to the Internet for anyone approaching a subject for the first time.

There are a number of gateways on nursing and related topics and the NHS site already noted (www.nhs.uk) is useful for access to health-care sites. In the UK, NMAP is an important gateway at www.nmap.ac.uk since it provides a 'guide to quality Internet resources in Nursing, Midwifery and the Allied Health Professions'. Links are provided via a 'query' box or through an 'advanced search' and, as in most gateways, there is a 'help' box available.

Referencing techniques

You should keep full reference details of each book or article consulted, in order to provide academic respectability and easy transfer of knowledge in the future. Referencing is discussed in detail in Chapter 6, but will be briefly summarised here.

If you reference a *book*, you require the following details:
- Author(s) surname(s) plus all initials
- Year of publication
- Complete title
- Edition number, if it is not the first edition
- Place of publication
- Publisher's name
- Note of series, if appropriate.

All this information can usually be found on the front and back of the title page. There are examples of references provided at the end of this chapter.

If you reference a *journal article* you require the following details:
- Author(s) surname(s) plus all initials
- Year of publication
- Title of article

- Name of journal
- Volume (and sometimes part) number
- Inclusive page numbers.

All this information can usually be found at the foot of each page, at the start of the article or on the contents page.

Referencing an item from an *electronic resource* is not straightforward (Kings College London 2002); however, items located via an online or CD-ROM source are of equal value to printed sources and should be referenced. To reference a full-text document from an online or CD-ROM database, you should include the standard aspects noted above but add a note 'Full-text (online)' and the date when the document was accessed. The reference to the Kings College London document given at the end of the chapter is a useful example. The college or institution that you use for your research will usually have a standard requirement for the layout of references and bibliography lists.

Over to you

Make up a 'dummy' reference card or computer file with the details of how you should record a journal reference, a book reference and an electronic resource reference.

Key points **Top tips**

Reference lists and bibliographies
- Reference lists are made up of items that you actually refer to and quote from in your document
- A bibliography is a list of material that you have not used directly but have found to be relevant to your theme and that helped form your opinions

The information search process

The emphasis throughout this chapter has been on sources of information and how you can access material needed for your studies. This can be summarised as follows.

- As you start looking for references, it is easier to begin with recent articles and books that summarise earlier work and theories. Literature review articles are useful, in that they summarise developments.
- Having noted your references, you should obtain the articles and books that are most appropriate from the libraries available to

you. Organise your references into some form of priority and check for those immediately available.

- If you are planning to use the interlibrary loan network, journal articles and books take time to arrive, so plan well ahead and allow plenty of time.
- Keep your options open and continue to note down new references and potential sources.
- Write down all relevant bibliographic details as well as the source of your information. This will save you time later on.
- Remember that your local librarians or information advisers are experts in finding and using information, and you should always ask for further help.

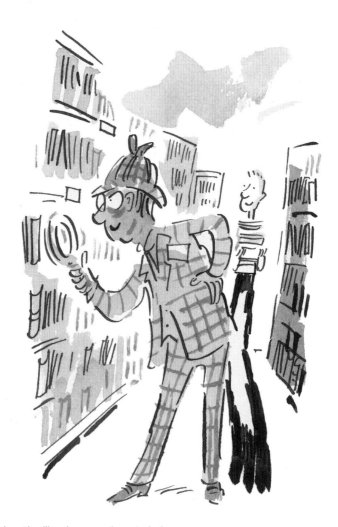

Remember, the librarians are there to help you.

Key points **Top tips**

To use library and information resources effectively:
● Clearly define your subject.
● Decide upon your searching strategy.
● Choose which libraries and information services are most appropriate and check if they are available to you.
● Decide which sources of information are most suitable for your needs.
● Begin your search, remembering to include full bibliographic details and record the source of your information.
● Obtain books, articles and other information.
● Read through all your gathered information and discard that which is not appropriate.

RRRRRRapid recap

Check your progress so far by working through each of the following questions.
1. List the points to consider before you start a search for information.
2. What benefits might LIS offer you?
3. What is a gateway or portal?

If you have difficulty with any of the questions, read through the section again to refresh your understanding before moving on.

References

Kings College London Information Services and Systems (2002) *Citing References* (online). Available at: www.kcl.ac.uk/iss (accessed 17.1.2003).

Marland, M. (1991) Skills of independence. *Education Guardian*, 20 October, 20.

4

Effective reading and note taking

Learning outcomes

By the end of this chapter you should be able to:

- Utilise the SQ3R method of reading material
- Know how to prioritise your reading
- Make effective notes when reading texts and during lectures.

Throughout your course you will need to read a great deal of material – some of which will be useful and some will not. It is, however, very frustrating to read every last word of a document or book and then discover that it is not useful. This is especially true if you have a lot of material to go through and only a limited amount of time in which to read it.

Another equally frustrating problem is when you 'read' a document through only to find that you have not been taking in what is written. This loss of concentration seems to occur more when we are tired but also tends to happen when the text is particularly difficult or tedious. Learning to be selective about what to read, learning to read quickly *and* being able to comprehend what is written are therefore important aspects of effective studying. This chapter looks at how you can develop a strategy for effective reading.

Prioritising reading material

You may find that, at times during your course, you are expected to do so much reading that you do not know where to start. Most lecturers will suggest reading material as a supplement to lectures and you may be required to read literature in order to complete assignments. From personal experience, I have found that it is often just not possible to read absolutely everything that is recommended and that the answer is to be selective and prioritise reading. Some lecturers produce long reading lists and don't give any indication of whether the items are essential or background reading. The first step is to ask for guidance. If you have a particularly heavy study schedule this will enable you to select the important texts you know you must read.

Secondly, you need to consult the notebook you were recommended in Chapter 1 to keep, which contains details of work to be completed, and identifies dates by which reading must be done. This should help you to prioritise reading and set deadlines for reading each text.

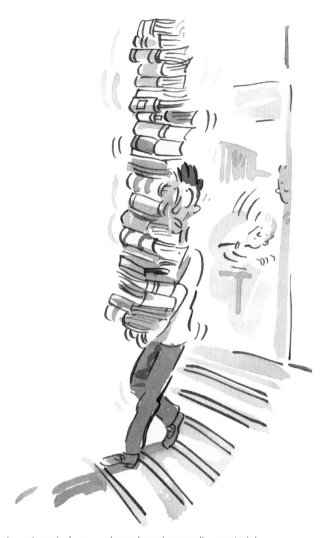

It is easy to get carried away when choosing reading material

Finally, when you have the chance but before the deadline for completing reading, take time to look at recommended (rather than essential) reading and note down the content of the text. You can do this very easily by taking brief notes from the abstract or summary in the case of a journal article, or from the index or contents page in the case of a book.

Effective reading

There may be times when you are given set or essential texts to read and you therefore have little choice but to sit down and read them. It is always a good idea to have pen and paper handy to make notes or, if the text is your own, you may prefer to use a highlighter pen to emphasise key points. Be careful not to overuse highlighter – I've seen many journal articles and books that have more highlighted sections than plain text. It is also unwise to highlight books or articles that you may use in the future for another purpose. It can be very frustrating to find that a book is full of highlighting of bits you are no longer interested in!

One system for effective reading is the SQ3R system, which is described below (SQ3R stands for Survey, Question, Read, Recall and Review).

S
Q
3
R

1. Survey

When you first pick up your text, do not be tempted to write anything until you have looked through or surveyed the whole text. It is always useful to start with the abstract or contents page/index. Then let your eyes run over the text, taking in headings, diagrams, tables and summarised sections. You should not read word-for-word at this stage.

2. Question

When you have finished surveying the text, sit back and reflect on what you have read and ask yourself certain questions. On your initial reading, try and put the text into the context of what you are studying. For example, if you are studying stigma in health care and are asked to read Stockwell's classic 1974 text *The Unpopular Patient* (an essential read for all aspiring health-care students), ask yourself how the text contributes to what you have already learned and decide which points you should be looking for within Stockwell's book. Students who are studying the text in relation to stigma will need to concentrate on different aspects of the work from students who are studying it in order to identify the methodologies used for the research.

When you have reflected on what you have read, ask yourself which parts of the text you need to re-read carefully and which parts you can safely re-survey. Write down your initial thoughts about important points. Finally, ask yourself if the text is really going to be helpful to you. If you decide it is, then go on to the next stage.

3. Read

The second time you go through the text, read more slowly but only read word-for-word the sentences or sections that are necessary to your work. If you cannot understand words, take time to look them up. Write the definitions down so that you do not forget them (self-adhesive notes are ideal for this purpose). Check that you are understanding what is written – most of us, at some time, have read something and have not taken in a word of it. Think carefully about the text and go back again to sentences that are confusing. If the sentence is long or contains, for example, double negatives, break it down into small parts to try and make sense of it. If you still find you cannot understand, then make a note to ask your subject lecturer for help.

4. Recall

When you have re-read and re-surveyed appropriate sections of the text, it is important that you again reflect on what you have read and put it into the context of what you are studying. This is important because the next stage involves making notes and you need to be absolutely clear that you have understood the text. If you have not understood it there is the danger that your notes will be inaccurate and will not reflect the text.

How often you stop to reflect will depend on your ability to concentrate and the nature of the text. Most books and articles, however, are written so that there are obvious stopping points. During the recall stage, summarise in brief note form the main points highlighted in the text and decide if there are areas you have not understood. Try re-reading confusing sections and go back to your brief notes to see if it now makes sense.

5. Review

Reviewing is the most important stage of SQ3R, because it helps to clarify ideas and ensures that you have not missed important points in the text. Reviewing involves going quickly through the process of survey, question, read and recall a second time – preferably after a break. It may seem tedious but is almost always worthwhile. If you have the time, it is better to leave the review for at least a day after reading. However, an hour or two is sufficient to be able to benefit from the last stage of the reading process.

Key points Top tips

- Ask for guidance from tutors when prioritising your reading material
- To read effectively, the easiest way is by using the SQ3R method

Note taking from texts

When you have read your text it may be appropriate to take notes either for future reference or for immediate use. If it is an article or book that you are going to keep, then notes can take the form of key headings and the appropriate page. If it is something you cannot keep, your notes will need to be more comprehensive. There are three stages to making notes from a written text.

1. Write down your own interpretation of what you have read. This will help you to remember what information you gathered and why it was important to you.

2. Carefully detail the main facts that may help you to remember the text. Write down main headings and important points as well as any related ideas. If you are taking notes in order to write an essay, you may wish to include some idea of when the information will be useful (introduction, section A, conclusion, etc.).

3. Write down other important information and/or quotations that you may need to refer to, with the appropriate page number. It is useful if you are reading a government report, for example, to write down the terms of reference or, if you are reading a research report, to write down the aims of the study. If you know you cannot keep the book or article, remember to note the full reference.

Key points **Top tips**

Taking notes from texts
- Keep a box of index cards, or set up a computer file, which indicates articles you have read and their key points.
- Create them using subject headings so that you build up your own resource box or file for future reference.

Note taking from lectures

Taking notes from a lecture serves three main purposes. They will:
- Help you to recall the lecture in future
- Help you to clarify the material discussed during the lecture
- Aid your concentration during the lecture.

Note taking from lectures involves different skills from note taking from reading material. Some lecturers make it very easy to take notes whereas others will not give you time to ask for clarification of points or take useful notes. It is important that you ascertain whether there are 'handouts' before you start to take notes. It is frustrating, to say the least, to spend time during a lecture taking careful notes only to be told at the end that the information is on a handout. You may also ask the lecturer – if you are not told – if you may ask questions during the lecture or if you should wait until the end.

When taking notes it is useful to develop your own shorthand. Miss out superfluous words such as 'the', 'and', 'but' etc. Try to be consistent with your abbreviations and shorthand. It may be months or years before you refer to something again and it is frustrating if you cannot understand your own notes.

If you miss a word or cannot understand something during the lecture then leave a dash and ask the lecturer to explain at the end. It is also a good idea to leave a margin as you can jot down related references and asterisk (*) those things that the lecturer tells you are important.

Read through your notes as soon as possible after the session and if necessary rewrite them to ensure that you have understood all the points (some students prefer to word process notes). This will help to reinforce what has been said in the lecture. If the lecture is one of a series by the same teacher, it is useful to read through your notes before the next session so that you can clarify with the lecturer confusing points arising from the previous lecture.

There are many ways of taking notes and it is worth experimenting to see which way suits your needs. The most usual three formats are summary, framework, and pattern.

Summary notes

Summary notes involve writing down, in a condensed form, the content of the lecture. The problem with this form of note taking is that you can become so intent on writing that you fail to listen and assimilate information effectively. In the past, as a way of trying to keep awake in exceptionally uninteresting lectures, I have made accurate summary notes. Unfortunately, I have little recollection of the actual lectures!

Framework notes

Framework notes are more difficult to make but are much less demanding in terms of concentration and time and are far easier to understand when you review them in the future.

Frameworking involves the use of letters, numbers, boxes, lists and diagrams. Main themes are underlined and subthemes are numbered. At the end of the lecture, go back and label main themes with letters, i.e. theme A, theme B, etc. The most important notes from the lecture can be boxed, in order to accentuate their importance.

Pattern notes

Patterning is usually only possible if you are familiar with the way the teacher delivers a lecture. The ideal type of session is where the lecturer starts with an overall topic heading and then expands. The topic would therefore be the core and the related points would branch out from the centre. In the example given in Figure 4.1, the centre theme of the lecture is 'study skills'.

Patterning can also be linear. In Figure 4.2, the theme of the lecture is 'effective reading and note taking'. Pattern notes are extremely useful for revision as they are easy to remember and follow logical thought patterns.

If you leave space between each note it will enable you to add related points or references later.

Over to you

- Try making summary, framework and pattern notes from a chapter in one of your course books.
- Decide which form of notes would be easier to remember, for instance for an exam, and which form enables you to reproduce the text accurately (try writing free text from your notes a week or two later).

Storing notes

Taking notes will be a waste of time if you never refer to them again. Their main purpose is to help you during the course but unless they are systematically filed you can waste valuable time trying to find them. Ring binders are still one of the most effective ways of filing notes and they are relatively inexpensive and easily stored. It is worth buying a separate binder for each major subject you are studying. Use dividing cards to separate subthemes within subject areas. It is better if you file notes as soon as possible after making them. I find it useful to stick a piece of lined paper on the inside of the ring binder to write down the contents. It can save time later on.

STUDY SKILLS
Organising Study (1)
Who?
What?
Why?
When?
Where?
How?
Information Technology (8)
CDROM/CAL
Spread sheets
Graphics
Database
WP
Output
Input
CPU
DTP
Library Skills (2)
Referencing
Libraries
Sources
Searching
Effective Reading (3)
S Q 3R
Cards
Notetaking (3)
Framework
Pattern
Summary
Evaluating Published Research (4)
Problem?
Literature?
Design?
Ethics?
Results?
Limitations?
Essay Writing (5)
Style
Layout
Content
Harvard
Vancouver
As (4)
Where
How
(6)
Projects
Seminars
Research Reports
(7) Examination Techniques
Diagrams
Themes
Title
Time
Aim
Preparation
Exam
Mindmaps
UKCC
Copyright (9)
1988 Act
Legal copies
Illegal copies
Permission

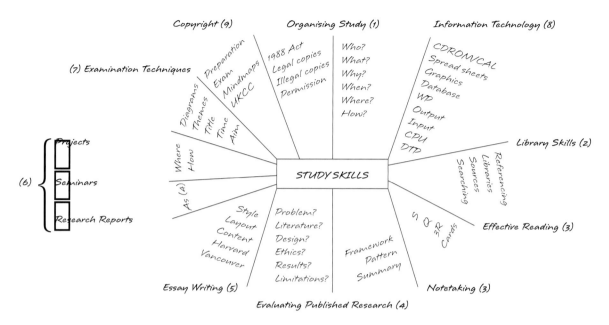

Figure 4.1 Patterning from a centre theme

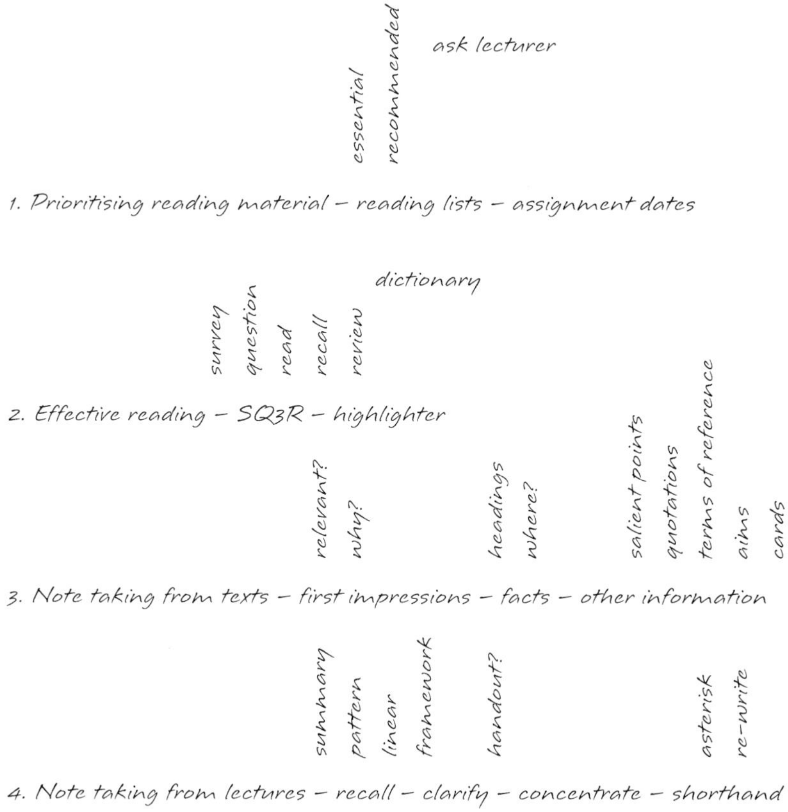

essential
recommended
ask lecturer
1. Prioritising reading material – reading lists – assignment dates
survey
question
read
recall
review
dictionary
2. Effective reading – SQ3R – highlighter
relevant?
why?
headings
where?
salient points
quotations
terms of reference
aims
cards
3. Note taking from texts – first impressions – facts – other information
summary
pattern
linear
framework
handout?
asterisk
re-write
4. Note taking from lectures – recall – clarify – concentrate – shorthand

Figure 4.2 Pattern lines

Key points | **Top tips**

Taking lecture notes

- If the teacher displays points on an overhead or data projector, it usually means those points are important so note them down. NB. Some teachers are prone to overusing projectors, in which case the above point will not apply!
- Always write down references and quotations (with page numbers if known). This will enable you to find out more information if you want to clarify points or widen your knowledge.
- Make notes of any part of the lecture that is accentuated or appears to be particularly important.
- Always read through your notes as soon as possible after a lecture. If the lecturer is a regular teacher, clarify confusing points at the earliest opportunity. If the lecturer is a guest speaker, ask the usual subject teacher or your personal tutor to clarify points for you.

RRRRRapid recap

Check your progress so far by working through each of the following questions.
1. What does SQ3R stand for?
2. What are the main aims of each (SQRRR)?
3. What are the 3 most common ways of note taking during lectures?
4. What must you always do as soon as possible after a lecture?

If you have difficulty with any of the questions, read through the section again to refresh your understanding before moving on.

References

Stockwell, F. (1974) *The Unpopular Patient*. Royal College of Nursing, London.

Further reading

Buzan, T. (2000) *Use Your Head* (Millennium edition). BBC Books, London.

Rowntree, D. (1998) *Learn How to Study*, 3rd edn. Time-Warner, London.

5

Evaluating and undertaking research

Learning outcomes

By the end of this chapter you should be able to:

- Understand why evaluating published research is valuable in your development as a health-care professional
- Ask yourself relevant questions to assist you when evaluating research
- Appreciate the different and most appropriate ways to carry out a particular research study
- Understand the ethical considerations of using people in your research and recognise the importance of gaining informed consent
- Interpret and evaluate the results of either your own research or someone else's.

All health-care professionals need to ensure that their practice is up-to-date and is based on the best available evidence. This means being able to read, understand, evaluate and utilise research. This is not easy as there are many different research approaches, methods and means of analysis and it is very difficult to become an expert in evaluating them all. Consequently utilisation of research by practising health-care professionals has been limited in many areas. There are three major reasons for this:

- Researchers tend to shroud their research in academic 'jargonese'
- They do not read research
- They do not have the skills to be able to evaluate research effectively.

This chapter looks at how to read and evaluate published research. This is a skill that is necessary for several reasons:

- You may be asked, as part of an assignment, to evaluate research
- If you undertake research as part of your course, evaluating other people's research will help you to clarify the direction of your own area of enquiry
- It will prepare you for using research in a practical way, to improve the quality of patient and client care.

Reading and evaluating research does require you to have some knowledge of research methodology and many pre- and postqualifying courses include research appreciation within the curriculum. However, there are different levels of evaluation and it is possible to assess some of the strengths and limitations of research by following a simple format. It is suggested, however, that before you start to evaluate research you ensure that you have a research methodology text (preferably one written for the profession you are training for) available for reference. There are many different texts available so before you buy one (and you really should consider buying, as you will find that it will be a useful purchase throughout your course and beyond) it is worth looking at a few in the library. Read the first chapter of a few to find one that you understand and that is written in a style you feel comfortable with. You will find a few useful texts in the Further Reading section at the end of this chapter.

Reading research

⊶ᴛ *Keywords*

....

SQ3R
Stands for Survey, Question, Read, Recall and Review and is an effective guide to follow when reading material

When you have gathered one or more pieces of research you should first of all decide whether it is going to be useful to you. The process of **SQ3R** (see Chapter 4) may help you decide. It will also familiarise you with the style of the researcher and the content and layout of the study.

If you decide that the research is useful there is a series of questions that you should attempt to answer. These are outlined in the Top Tips feature below. While you are reading the research study, it is useful to have a notebook and pencil to hand so that you can write down the relevant answers.

Introduction and the problem studied

Researchers will usually 'set the scene' for their enquiry by defining the problem that led them to undertake the research and giving a rationale (the reason) for the study. Ask yourself if the problem seems important. Some researchers will outline the purpose of their enquiry, research questions, objectives and/or a hypothesis within this introductory section. It is, however, more usual for these to be detailed following the literature review, as one of the main purposes of searching the literature is to enable researchers to refine their ideas and increase their knowledge of the subject being studied.

Literature review

All research studies should review other research and literature that relates to their identified problem. Reviewing literature identifies what research has already been done in a particular field and helps to shape the researcher's ideas. It is worth mentioning at this point, however, that some researchers undertaking some qualitative forms of research (usually phenomenology and grounded theory) do not fully review the literature prior to undertaking their data collection because they do not want to have preconceived ideas that might influence or bias their work.

Top tips

When reading a literature review as part of a research study, you need to ask several questions:

- Is the literature relevant to the study?
- How old is the literature? If it is old, does it matter?
- Does the researcher use literature from one country or from many countries? Does it matter?
- Is the literature described or does the researcher attempt to review each piece of literature and discuss its strengths and weaknesses in relation to the other literature reviewed?
- Does the researcher discuss the implications of the literature?
- Are the sources of the literature used clearly documented?

Research aims, questions, objectives and hypotheses

Following the literature review and before the methodology section of the research report, the researcher should clearly identify the purpose of the study. This will include setting out the broad aims of the study and may involve the identification of a number of questions that the researcher wishes to answer and/or objectives they set out to achieve. As a result of the questions or objectives, a hypothesis may or may not be formulated. A hypothesis is a statement that the researcher sets out either to support or reject. An example is given in the case study of Sinead's research question.

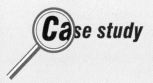
Case study

Sinead's research question

Sinead is a ward sister and has identified that student nurses who work more than 7 days without a day off tend to have an increase in sickness. She wants to formally research this with the aim of discovering whether working 7 days or more without a break increases sickness rates. She could express this as a question: 'Do student nurses who work more than 7 days without a break have an increased sickness rate?' Alternatively she could turn her question into a hypothesis or statement: 'Student nurses who work 7 days or more without a break have increased sickness'.

The use of questions and/or hypotheses will depend upon how Sinead decides to investigate the problem. This is discussed more fully later in the chapter.

Sample

When the researcher starts to plan research, decisions have to be made about how the problem is to be investigated and how many people or subjects need to be involved in order to achieve the aims of the research. The researcher should state how many people or subjects were involved and how they were chosen to participate in the study. Some researchers will study an entire population (the total number of people who could potentially be included) and others will study a sample proportion of the population. The researcher should outline a justification for using a sample and it is usual for researchers to set out clear criteria for sample selection. If the subjects within a defined sample refuse to participate, the researcher should refer to the number(s) of such subjects involved, and similarly if subjects withdraw after the study is under way. If the researcher used a questionnaire, the response rate should be clearly stated.

If a sample is used you need to decide if the people within the sample are representative of the total potential population.

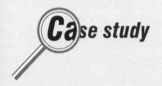

Case study

Sanjeev's research study

Sanjeev is a student nurse and wants to undertake a study of student sickness rates at the hospital at which he is on placement. For the purposes of his study, the total population would be the total number of students in training at that hospital. If there were 200 students, he could decide that, rather than include everyone, a proportion of the total should be studied. How he chooses that proportion is vitally important to his study. He could choose a sample of 50 students at random, so that every student has an equal chance of being included in the study. If his choice is random, the sample should be representative of the population and implications drawn from the results can be applied to the total student population. If, however, he decides to choose a sample including 50 first-year students, their sickness patterns may not be representative of those of second and third-year students. The implications of his study could not therefore be applied to second- and third-years.

If the researcher is undertaking an experiment, which usually involves manipulation of one group of subjects and comparing the effects of the manipulation against a second un-manipulated group known as the *control group*, it is important to ascertain how the researcher assigned subjects to each group. A further example is given in the case study opposite.

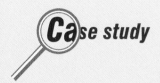

Case study

Stuart's experiment

Stuart has just entered nurse training and has chosen to set up an experiment for his research study. He is interested in looking at the effects of night duty on sickness rates, so it will be necessary for him to compare sickness of students doing night duty with those doing day duty. He needs to select two groups of students that are similar with the only definable difference being that one group does night duty and one group does not. He knows that the students should be at the same stage of training and that their assignment to the night duty or day duty groups should be random, so that each student has an equal chance of being placed in either group.

If, for example, he compared first-year students who only do day duty with third-year students who do night duty, the results could be attributed to reasons other than the manipulation (in this case, night duty).

Ethical considerations

Research involving people is governed by codes that are designed to protect them and ensure that they do not suffer physical, psychological or social harm. Researchers should always consider the ethics of their research and, if necessary, should obtain permission from appropriate bodies. Health-care professionals undertaking research on patients, on patient records or on NHS property must always consult the ethics committee, and should state within the study that they have done so. The appropriate managers should also be consulted and their permission obtained.

The subjects involved in research should normally have the opportunity to give their *informed consent* or to refuse to participate. Informed consent can only be given by subjects if they have received information relating to the purpose of the study, what they will be required to do if they agree to participate and what will happen to the results of the study. They should also be informed as to whether they will be identified or if their responses will be anonymous and regarded as confidential. Details of explanations given to subjects should be clearly documented in the study.

Subjects should be allowed to withdraw their consent any time during the enquiry.

Keywords

Qualitative
Describing the quality or features of something

Quantitative
Describing the number or quantity of something

Methodology

There are two major approaches to research; **qualitative** and **quantitative**. Most research books include discussions about both, and indicate the sorts of problems that would usually be studied quantitatively and those that would usually be studied qualitatively.

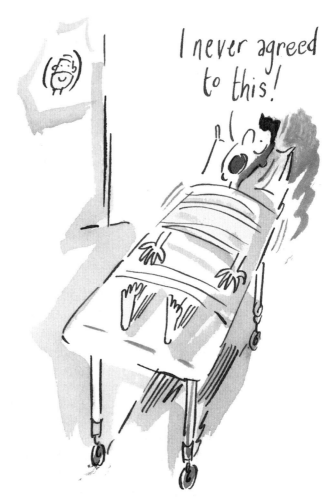

Always ensure that your research subjects are fully briefed on what's involved in the study

Depending on the approach used, the researcher will use various *data collection instruments* in order to gather the information required to achieve the aims of the study, answer research questions, meet objectives and support or reject the hypothesis, if there is one. Data collection instruments include self-report measures (such as interviews, questionnaires), biophysical measures (such as thermometers, blood analysis, tape measures), observation schedules, etc. The researcher should state why a particular measure has been chosen and you should ask yourself whether the instrument used is appropriate.

The use of data collection instruments is important when evaluating research. Many researchers use previously tried and tested instruments (such as anxiety scales, visual analogue scales, attitude measures, etc.) and they should state who designed the instrument, the context in which it has been used and how they have ensured that it is consistently reliable in measuring what it intends to measure. If the researcher designs a new data collection instrument, e.g. a questionnaire or attitude scale, it should be tested to ensure that it is reliable. This is done through a variety of ways, such as undertaking a **pilot study.**

If a pilot study has been undertaken the researcher should state how this was carried out and give the results. If any changes have been made as a result of the pilot study, these should be clearly stated.

Finally it is worth mentioning that some researchers use a variety of data collection instruments to answer a single research question as this can enhance the validity of the research.

Results of the study

The results of the study should be reported clearly and presented in a logical way. If tables, graphs or charts are used they should be easily understood and should be applicable to the study. Chapter 7 discusses appropriate ways of presenting numerical data.

Any statistical processes or tests used to analyse and describe data and/or test hypotheses should be explained and the observed values and the level of **probability** stated. A knowledge of statistics is valuable when evaluating research in order to judge if the right statistical test has been used and if errors have been made. The Further Reading section at the end of this chapter gives useful references.

Following the results section, the researcher should discuss and interpret the findings. Results should be discussed in relation to the purpose of the study, the research questions, objectives and the hypothesis (if applicable). It is also usual to refer back to the literature review, where relevant. The purpose of this section of the research report is to compare and contrast the results of the new research with previous work in the field. It is worth noting that some qualitative researchers combine their results and discussion into one, rather than two separate, sections.

The researcher should then highlight any limitations of the research. For example, if the response rate to a questionnaire was very low, it could have yielded **atypical** data that would influence the findings.

Most (but not all) research will have implications for practice and the researcher should discuss these fully. As a result of the study, the

Keywords

Pilot study
A trial run of the research using a small sample

Keywords

Probability
The extent to which something is likely to happen

Keywords

Atypical
Not typical or usual

researcher will also make recommendations, which should relate to the results. In addition, the researcher may suggest areas where future research is needed. It should be remembered that a great deal of research actually raises more questions than it answers. Finally, the researcher should draw together the study with a conclusion although some researchers will place the conclusion prior to the recommendations.

Overall impressions

Following your evaluation of research, it is always worth reflecting on the study as a whole and asking a few questions.

- Was the study readable and interesting?
- Did it really achieve its purpose?
- Did it include any irrelevant material?
- Does it contribute to existing knowledge?

Key points | **Top tips**

When evaluating research:

- Read the research study through, following the SQ3R system before you start to evaluate it formally.

- Design a numerical coding system for undertaking your evaluation. Published research (especially when it is presented as a summary) can appear muddled and may not follow a logical format. Using a code can clarify points for you. For example, label stated problems as (1), literature review as (2), research questions/objectives as (3), and so on.

- If you are comparing the results of two or more studies, use different-coloured highlighter pens to accentuate related points. For example, if study A discussed the beneficial effects of using dressing X on leg ulcers, study B found that dressing X made no significant difference and study C found that dressing X delayed healing, highlight them all in the same colour so that when you come to write about dressing X you can easily find the appropriate sections in all three studies.

- Remember that, even if a piece of research is not useful for a particular assignment, it may be relevant in the future. Make up a card with the full reference and a brief description of the study and file it, or add it to you computer file.

RRRRRRapid recap

Check your progress so far by working through each of the following questions.

1. List six things to look for in a literature review.
2. What are the two major *approaches* to research?
3. What is the purpose of undertaking a pilot study?
4. List four questions you might ask yourself about your overall impressions of a research study.

If you have difficulty with any of the questions, read through the section again to refresh your understanding before moving on.

Further reading

Grbich, C. (1998) *Qualitative Research in Health: An introduction*. Sage, London.

Greig, A. and Taylor, J. (1998) *Doing Research with Children*, Sage, London.

Jordan, K., Ong, B.N. and Croft, P. (1998) *Mastering Statistics: A guide for health service professionals and researchers*. Nelson Thornes, Cheltenham.

O'Dochartaigh, N. (2002) *The Internet Research Handbook*. Sage, London.

Walsh, M. and Wigens, L. (2003) *Introduction to Research*. Nelson Thornes, Cheltenham.

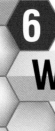

6

Writing essays and reports, and referencing

Most people have had to write essays or reports at some time during their lives, but fully referenced, research-based, academic essays and reports can present difficulties for many students. This chapter looks at how to write academic essays, how to structure reports and how to accurately reference your work. The information given here aims to help you with your essay and report writing but you should always check the guidelines for each assignment with your lecturer for the precise requirements.

Essay writing

Essay writing is never easy and can be extremely time-consuming. The content of an essay is what will gain you the majority of your marks but the presentation of the material will help to create a favourable impression and will assist the lecturer to assess your understanding and interpretation of a subject. With badly presented work, there is also the danger that the lecturer will not actually be able to read or interpret what has been written, so marks will undoubtedly be lost. It is worth checking with the lecturer who will be assessing your work what percentage of marks, if any, will be assigned for presentation. While you should always aim to hand in carefully written work, a knowledge of how marks are weighted will help you to know what the lecturer is expecting. Most universities will provide this sort of information as standard practice in student handbooks. These should also provide you with the criteria for assessment so that you know from the outset what you need to produce in order to pass the assessment. Some universities take this even further and will outline the criteria for a minimum pass through to a distinction.

The following section looks at how to lay out essays and discusses the content and style of academic prose.

Layout

There are several things you can do to ensure that your essay is correctly set out. Essays should always contain an introduction, a 'middle bit' and a conclusion. They may or may not make recommendations. Content is discussed in the next section.

Before you start to write your essay you should check with your lecturer:

- Does the essay have to be typed or can you write it out? If typed, are there any stipulations about line spacing, e.g. double spacing?
- Can you write on both sides of the paper?
- What referencing style should you use?
- What information should you include on the title page, e.g. name or examination number, date, institution?
- Do you need to leave margins on one or both sides of the pages?
- Are there any other guidelines?

In addition to these points there are several basic things you can do to make your work more aesthetically pleasing.

Quotations

If you need to quote directly from a published work it looks neater if the quote is slightly indented. You should always start on a new line when you begin the quotation and recommence text on a new line. The text should be quoted word for word and the page number should be included. For example:

> Buzan (2000) discusses that the brain is able to sort information that is non-linear, a point that has been recently confirmed by other research:
>
> > 'Your brain's non-linear character is further confirmed by recent biochemical, physiological and psychological research. Each area of research is discovering to its amazement and restrained delight that the brain is not only non-linear but is so complex and interlinked that it guarantees centuries of exhilarating research and exploration' (p. 96).
>
> In practical terms the brain can sort such information as photographs . . . .

Diagrams

If you include diagrams, tables or graphs you should allow adequate room so that they do not appear to be cluttered. Diagrams should be clearly labelled and should appear with relevant portions of text. For further information on this, see Chapter 7.

Content

Most of the essays you are asked to write will involve studying the literature and writing about it. The flow chart in Figure 6.1 outlines the process of organising your essay writing:

The first stage is to gather literature and other material from appropriate sources (Chapter 3 gives information on literature searching). Read through literature as you obtain it and make notes about which section of the essay it will be appropriate for. If it is your own book, highlighter pens can be useful for marking relevant parts of the text. Discard material that will not be used but, if you feel it may be appropriate at a later stage, make up an index card with the bibliographic details and a summary of the material, or create a computer file.

The next stage is to draft an essay plan, which should be checked, if possible, with your lecturer, or if not with a colleague. When you have done this, you can start to write your essay. If you

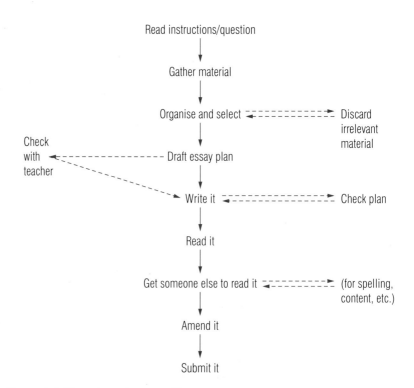

Figure 6.1 *Flow chart of essay writing process*

prefer to write by hand initially, it is worth leaving a bit of space under each paragraph at this stage so that you can add in further information if necessary. It is always difficult to calculate your wordage so clearly separating paragraphs will enable you to identify areas where you can add or subtract words. Obviously, word processing your work from the start makes this whole process much easier.

After you have written your first draft, read it and ask someone else to read it. I always ask a lecturer or colleague to read work at this stage, although some universities have regulations prohibiting lecturers from reading drafts. It is also worth asking someone who knows nothing about the subject to read it. You then have the benefit of someone who is able to judge the content as well as someone who can correct grammar and flow. Make any necessary amendments on your rough draft and re-read it. It is sometimes useful to read it out loud and record it on to a tape. Both as you record it and when listening back, you will soon pick up repetitive words and sentences as well as confusing passages. When reading into a tape recorder, ignore anything in brackets and this will tell you if you are referencing correctly.

Over to you

Try reading the sentences below out loud remembering to ignore anything in brackets:

1. (Jones, 2002) states that there is nothing worse than trying to understand long and tortuous sentences.
2. Jones (2002) states that there is nothing worse than trying to understand long and tortuous sentences.
3. There is nothing worse than trying to understand long and tortuous sentences Jones (2002).
4. There is nothing worse than trying to understand long and tortuous sentences (Jones, 2002).

Hopefully you will have decided that 1 and 3 don't make sense and are incorrectly referenced!

The final stage is to write for submission. Don't forget to photocopy your work, as lecturers have been known to lose assignments! Universities require you to submit typed essays throughout your course and a word processor will save you an enormous amount of time, especially when it comes to amending text. It will also check spelling and grammar and count words. If someone else is typing your work, allow yourself time to read it through and have it amended if necessary.

It has already been mentioned that essays should have an introduction, a middle bit and a conclusion. The following section outlines the principles of what you should include in which bit.

The introduction

This should give an overview of the subject and outline the points that you are going to discuss in your essay. It is often useful to start your essay by restating the question in the form of a statement and then take the major areas for discussion from the wording of the statement. Do not include in your introduction things that are irrelevant or that you are not going to expand on.

You may feel you wish to rationalise your approach to the subject and it may be appropriate to define certain issues. For example, if you are writing an essay about health education you might give a definition of what health education is.

The 'middle bit'

This is where you discuss the main themes that you have already mentioned in the introduction. There may be one theme that has different aspects to it or there may be several themes. If you can, allow your 'middle bit' to develop logically and link areas if possible. It is usual to start with general issues and progress to more specific areas. If there is only one theme, the general issues would be discussed in early paragraphs and more specific issues later. If there are several themes and each theme takes the form of a paragraph, the beginning sentences should be general with more specific information closing the paragraph.

The conclusion

Here, you draw your work to a close. It should contain the major points in a summarised form and refer back to the original question. In addition, as a result of the essay, you may be asked to make recommendations. Do not, however, make recommendations about things that you have not discussed. Your conclusion should not introduce any new ideas but you may highlight areas that you feel need further study.

It is always worth making it clear when your conclusion is beginning. One way of doing this is to start your conclusion with 'To conclude . . .'.

Style

Many students find it difficult to write essays in an academic style and it takes practice and discipline to produce work that is not 'journalistic'. Some assessors will allow students to write in the first person but many will not. With thought, you can write in the third person without too much difficulty. Two examples are given below, the first written in the first person and second written in the third person:

- **Example 1**: During this essay I will discuss three factors which can influence health. The factors I have chosen are diet, smoking and sexuality.

- **Example 2**: During this essay, three factors which can influence health are discussed. These factors are diet, smoking and sexuality.

Another common problem with style is the use of sexist language (Eichler 1988, Kirkman 1992). This is apparent in four forms:

- Using male terms for generic purposes, e.g. 'man is a complex being'

- Use of non-parallel terms, e.g. 'a man and his wife'

- Consistently naming one sex before another, e.g. 'he/she'

- Using generic terms when referring to one sex, e.g. referring to 'parents' when only discussing mothers.

As with eliminating first-person terminology, getting rid of sexist language is not usually difficult. Two further examples are given below; the first includes sexist language and the second does not.

- **Example 1**: During the admission interview the nurse should ensure that she allows time for the patient to ask questions. If the patient is confused it may be necessary to ask one of his/her relatives to confirm details.

- **Example 2**: During the admission interview the nurse should allow time for the patient to ask questions. If the patient is confused it may be necessary to ask a relative to confirm details.

Another common problem is writing at an academic level below that which is required. For example, your work might be too descriptive or not sufficiently analytical. Most universities will produce what they call **level descriptors**.

The Quality Assurance Agency (www.qaa.ac.uk) has produced the Framework for Higher Education Qualifications and it is worth consulting this if your University does not provide specific guidance (QAA 2001).

The most difficult leap you may experience is making the transition between writing at academic levels 1, 2 and 3. At

⚷ *Keywords*

Level descriptors
The general requirements of what universities expect to see in work at first-, second- and third-year undergraduate level, master's level, etc.

level 1 it is expected that work will be largely descriptive, at level 2 your work should demonstrate analysis and at level 3 critical analysis. Below are examples of writing at the three different levels.

Description: (level 1 skill)
Nurses frequently fail to utilise research in their practice (Funk et al 1993).

Analysis: (level 2 skill)
Funk et al (1993), in a study of research utilisation in the USA, found that nurses frequently fail to utilise research in their practice. The study took a random sample of nurses from the US register of nurses and administered a 33-item structured questionnaire that yielded numerical data. These data highlighted the main barriers and facilitators to research utilisation.

Critical analysis: (level 3 skill)
Funk et al (1993), in a study of research utilisation in the USA, found that nurses frequently fail to utilise research in their practice. The study took a random sample of nurses from the US register of nurses and administered a 33-item structured questionnaire that yielded numerical data. These data highlighted the main barriers and facilitators to research utilisation. The study by Funk et al was strengthened by the rigorous testing of the barrier and facilitator scales used. However, the findings must be reviewed with caution in applying them to the UK because the sample comprised only nurses in the USA, who undertake different initial training. Polit and Hungler (1997) suggest that the findings of any study can only be generalised (external validity) to those who had an equal chance of being included in the sample. A further study that did address this issue was undertaken by Walsh (1997), who found that similar results could be generalised across groups of nurses in the UK. His results were very similar to Funk's but were in contrast to . . .

A useful and simple example of differentiating between academic levels can be found in the following comparison.

If you take a bowl of fruit containing apples, oranges and one lemon you might describe it as follows:

There were two apples, which are round and green, three oranges, which are round and orange, and one lemon, which is yellow and oval in shape.

You might then analyse:

> When the fruit is cut open it is possible to see that the oranges and lemon are similar, in that they are segmented, whereas the apple has a smooth texture with an inner core containing pips.

You might critically analyse by adding to the above:

> When the fruit is cut open it is possible to see that the oranges and lemon are similar in that they are segmented whereas the apple has a smooth texture with an inner core containing pips. The apple can be eaten without removing the peel and there is evidence to suggest that the peel has a higher fibre content than the flesh inside (Greenfinger 1992), making apples a healthy eating option. The orange and lemon should be peeled before being eaten. Citrisini (1984) suggests that lemons . . .

Some key words/phrases you might consider including, which might help to make you think about critical analysis are:

- In contrast . . .
- Conversely . . .
- Therefore, in addition to . . . .

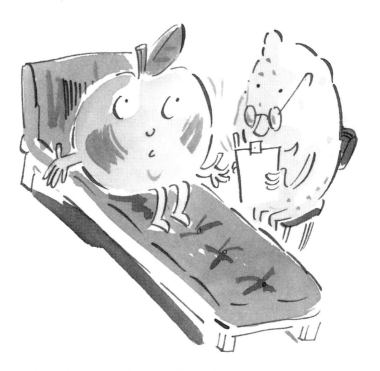

Using analysis takes your work on to a deeper level

Report writing

You may be required as part of an assessment to produce a report.

Theory and practice

There are many different reasons why reports are produced in real life situations – usually to inform decision-making processes but also for incidents such as accidents, critical events, etc. One of the more usual reasons for producing a report is to present a research study.

You should be given guidelines relating to the expected content and some indication is usually made in relation to the word limit. It is not within the remit of this book to look at how to undertake research. Mark Walsh and Lynne Wigens cover this in detail in another book in the *Foundations in Nursing and Health Care* series, *Introduction to Research*. It is worth noting that many students have lost valuable marks because they have presented their research incorrectly and the aim of this section is to describe one of the usual formats for writing a research report and how to present statistical information.

Reports tend to be much more concise, factual and structured than essays, and as such require careful planning about how you can logically portray your ideas. As a rough guide, research reports usually comprise a number of parts.

Title page

Keep this simple, with a title that reflects the nature of the report. Include information as required, such as your student number, name, etc.

Acknowledgements

Most research reports involve other people, whether it be a statistician who has helped you to analyse your data, a friend who typed it for you or your family who have been forced to eat their meals on trays for 6 months because you took over the dining table! It is usual to acknowledge such help. It is, however, possible for an acknowledgement list to get out of hand so try to limit thanks to those who made essential contributions (or sacrifices!). Thanking the family dog for his patience over the lack of walks over the last 6 months is a bit over the top!

A summary (or abstract)

This should be able to be used independently of the full report. It should contain the key recommendations and should include nothing that cannot be found in your actual report. The summary should not normally exceed more that 10% of the length of the full report. Check whether or not it counts towards the word limit of the assignment, if there is one. The summary is sometimes produced as a list of bullet points or short sentences. An example of this can be found at the beginning of every chapter in this book. You cannot produce the summary until after you have written the full report. I try to produce a short SWOT (strengths, weaknesses, opportunities and threats) table at the end of each section of a report, detailing its contents, and I build up the summary from these. That way I can ensure that the summary contains a balance of points and gives the reader a 'taster' of the full nature of the report.

Contents list

This should give the main themes of the study with appropriate page numbers. You may also give a list of tables and appendices. Complete this when you have finished the report.

An introduction

Just like the introduction to an essay, this should clearly set out what you have done and how you have done it. It should set the scene for the study and include information about how the study originated, why it is being undertaken, the significance of the problem or issue being investigated and what the research expects to contribute to existing knowledge.

Literature review

A literature review involves selecting appropriate references and providing an analytical and critical evaluation. It is usual to review literature of a general nature before that which is more specific. All literature should be relevant to the problem being studied and linked to the problem where appropriate. Any implications drawn should be clearly stated. The views of the authors whose literature is reviewed should be compared and contrasted. Remember to properly reference all the sources you have used.

A final point about literature is to remember to include classic works. Further information about literature searching is given in Chapter 3.

The theoretical or conceptual framework

Research is undertaken in order to add to, or strengthen, an existing body of knowledge. In some cases this may mean generating a new theory that can later be tested or it may mean testing an existing theory, which you will strengthen through your findings or question if your findings differ.

In some types of research (typically phenomenology, ethnography and grounded theory) the researcher deliberately avoids theoretical propositions at the outset of the enquiry. For other types of qualitative and quantitative designs, theory development as part of the design phase is essential whether the purpose is further theory development or theory testing. The researcher may, for example, undertake research into the effects of extended prescribing on the nurse's role, which will add specific knowledge in that field. It might also add to a broader body of knowledge about professionalism or the progress of change in nursing depending on the focus of the study. In this example, professionalism or change might be the underlying theory and the more specific study of extended prescribing is further developing the theory. A theoretical framework therefore provides a context for examining a problem. A common error made by students is that they describe a particular framework and it then gets 'lost'. The framework should provide a basis for observations, research designs and interpretations. It places the research problem in a theoretical context, bringing meaning to the problem and the findings.

The purpose

After the literature review the purpose of the study should be clearly stated. This can take the form of research aims, research questions, research objectives and/or a research hypothesis. If there is more than one they should be placed in order of priority. Questions, objectives and hypotheses should be concise and specific.

Methodology

Firstly, the population(s) or sample(s) used for the study should be described, giving details of numbers used and the characteristics of subjects, e.g. 50 children admitted to hospital for routine minor surgical procedures or 30 nurses undertaking a postregistration degree in nursing. You should justify both the numbers used and the characteristics. Sampling techniques should be clearly defined and the type of sample stated, e.g. random sample, convenience sample, cluster sample, etc.

If questionnaires are used the response rate obtained should be stated. If the response rate is low you will need to reflect that the sample may be atypical and remember to discuss the effects within the limitations section of the study.

Secondly, the research design should be discussed with details about how validity is to be upheld. The data collection instruments should be discussed in detail and, if appropriate, included as an appendix to the study. If a data collection instrument designed by another researcher is used, details of its use and reliability, as well as

○━π Keywords

Variables
Factors within a research study that can influence results – for example, marital status is a social variable

○━π Keywords

Null hypothesis
A testable statement that is either supported or rejected through the research process

appropriate references, should be given. Details about how **variables** are controlled and measured should be given.

Finally, ethical considerations should be discussed and you should state what you perceive as being the major ethical issues and how you handled them. Your discussion should give details including information given to subjects, permission sought and obtained and any other related information. It should be made clear exactly what the subjects needed to do within the study.

Pilot study

It is not always necessary to carry out a pilot study. However, if you have designed your own research tools or amended those of someone else, you may need to undertake a pilot study in order to evaluate the reliability of your data collection instruments (see Walsh and Wigens (2003) for a comprehensive discussion on evaluating reliability). There are certain protocols that should be followed when testing the reliability of tools and these should be described in this section. If amendments need to be made as a result of the pilot study, they should be clearly stated.

Results

The results of the study should be presented in a value-free way. If statistical tests are used they should be clearly explained and observed values and probability levels given. You should indicate if levels of statistical significance obtained are sufficient to reject your **null hypothesis**.

It is acceptable to report numbers within the text but if you start a sentence with a number you should write it in full. For example:

> Forty one percent of respondents replied Yes and 59% replied No to question 4, which asked if they felt that smoking should be banned from all forms of public transport.

Information given in diagrammatic form should be clearly labelled and interspersed with relevant written text. It is rarely necessary to present data both diagrammatically and within the text but more usual to state that the results of a particular question are given in Table X. Table and figure numbers should always be in sequence as they appear in the text. Further information about presenting statistical data is given in the following section.

Discussion

Following the value-free reporting of results, a discussion should be included where you can interpret your data. During your discussion you should link results back to your research aims, questions, objectives and hypotheses (if applicable). It may also be appropriate to refer back to your literature review. For example, if your findings uphold or contrast with the findings of previous research, you should discuss possible reasons for these similarities or differences.

Limitations of your research should also be discussed at this point, including failure to control or identify variables, sampling issues, reliability of data collection instruments and external validity.

Recommendations

Most research will have implications. These may include the need to change current practice or could suggest areas where further study is necessary, perhaps with a larger sample in a wider setting. A great deal of research will raise more questions than it answers and some will not have any implications at all. Try not to be disappointed if you do not achieve the results you anticipated. If you have followed the correct protocol your research will still be valuable. Some of the most interesting research I have undertaken has failed to support a hypothesis but has led to further research because of the data yielded.

Conclusion

Your conclusion should pull together the main points from your research and summarise the study. Its value in relation to change should be discussed with brief reference to noted limitations. It is usual to make a final statement linking your findings with your research aims, questions, objectives or hypotheses.

References

A list of references should be included either in numerical order (the Vancouver style) or in alphabetical order (the Harvard style). Full details of referencing are given later in this chapter.

Bibliography or further reading

A list of reference sources used but not cited within the text may be included after the reference list. Some universities allow students to combine reference and bibliography lists and you should therefore seek clarification from your lecturer.

Appendices

Appendices are included, if relevant, at the end of the report. Information included does not normally count towards the overall word limit of the project (check this with your lecturer), and can include supporting information, models, printed extracts, data collection instruments, etc. Appendices should be numbered with roman numerals, i.e. I, II, III, IV, and a list of appendices should be included, giving the number and the content.

Presenting statistical information

Data can be presented in the form of tables, graphs and charts, which can give added visual impact to the text, as well as reducing the wordage. The following section discusses the appropriate presentation of statistical information as an alternative to written text.

Tables

Tables are the most straightforward way of presenting statistical information and have the advantage that percentages and/or raw data can be easily seen.

It is important, however, that tables are not confusing and can be read without difficulty. Tables should only contain information that is relevant but should contain enough information for the reader to be able to understand what is being presented without needing to refer back to the text. Each table should be clearly labelled and the source of the information given if appropriate. An example is given in Table 6.1.

Line graphs

Line graphs are very useful for showing trends and should enable the reader to understand relevant information easily. Line graphs have an x and a y axis (the x axis is the horizontal axis). The x axis usually indicates the time scale (e.g. a year). As with tables, line graphs must be clearly labelled and particular attention should be paid to scales used. The reader should also be able to work out the exact figures from the graph so information relating to frequency scales should be clear (e.g. 1000s). Each point on the scale should be equal. An example is given in Figure 6.2.

Bar charts

Bar charts are ways of showing frequencies for discontinuous categories. Each chart should be clearly labelled and the reader

Table 6.1 Admissions to Ward 4 by diagnosis and age in July

	Age group (years)				
	<1	1–3	4–7	8–11	>11
Infectious diseases	14	11	7	6	4
Respiratory	26	19	11	9	9
Surgical	17	16	25	28	14
Malignant	1	2	6	7	4
Burns	2	4	1	2	1
Fracture	1	0	2	6	21
Total	**61**	**52**	**52**	**58**	**53**

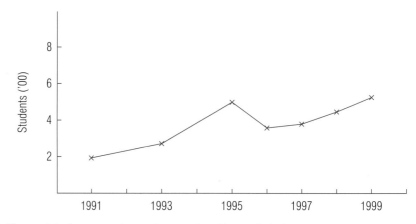

Figure 6.2 *Pass rates for students undertaking statistical evaluation 1991–99*

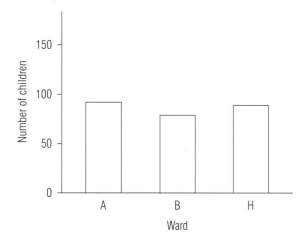

Figure 6.3 *Bar chart showing admission rates of children during June 2002*

should be able to interpret the data easily. Bar charts can be drawn either horizontally or vertically. An example is given in Figure 6.3.

Histograms

Histograms are bar charts that represent continuous data and are therefore useful for indicating trends. The principles of using line graphs apply to histograms. Again, each chart must be clearly labelled and scale is very important. Figure 6.4 provides an example of a histogram.

Pie charts

A pie chart is another way of presenting statistical information visually and is a circle where 360° is used to represent 100% of a sample. It is still important that the reader can work out exact figures from the information given and the charts should be labelled accurately.

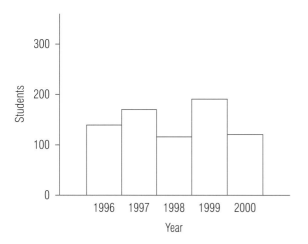

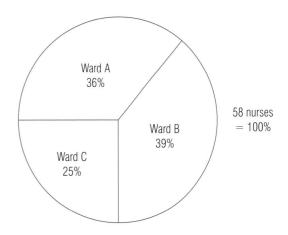

Figure 6.4 *Number of student passes in physiotherapy*   **Figure 6.5** *Distribution of staff in surgery unit*

One problem with pie charts is that there is a limit to the number of divisions that can be made in the pie without it becoming very difficult to interpret. The suggested maximum number of divisions is eight. An example of a pie chart is given in Figure 6.5.

Key points **Top tips**

When writing a research report:

● Remember that a report is usually being written to inform a decision-making process or to record critical events. It should therefore be a factual, descriptive document.

● The summary should not contain any additional information to that found in the main body of text. You will find it easier to write the summary last, even though it will appear at the beginning of your report.

● Find a finished report similar to the one you're writing and use it as a template for the structure of yours.

● Remember that it may be important to present some of your data in a visual way.

● Statistical data is often better presented in the form of a table, graph or chart.

Over to you

Find a research report in a journal and identify the stages of the research process used by the researcher(s).

Referencing

Referencing work correctly is vitally important as it tells the assessor where you have found your information, how up to date it is and if it is appropriate to your essay. If necessary, the references enable them to go to the source of your information to read the work at first hand. It also helps the assessor to differentiate between your personal thoughts and experiences and those of others.

There are two basic styles of referencing, described below, although you will find variations in some journals and textbooks. Both styles are acceptable academically; however, you should not mix styles. Some universities will specify the use of one particular style and individual lecturers may express a preference. You will need to check before you start to write your assignment. Most universities will provide guidance on their referencing style in student handbooks or in their libraries.

The Vancouver system

The Vancouver style is also referred to as the numerical system. The *Nursing Times*, for example, uses this system and it involves the use of numbers within the text that are cross-referenced at the end of the essay. For example:

> Children should be accompanied by their parents when they stay in hospital[1,2] although it is generally thought that as they get older they are better able to deal with their experiences.[3,4]

References 1,2, etc. are given in full in the reference list as follows:

1. Jones J. Children in hospital. *Nursing Times* 1990; **85**(15): 14.
2. Taylor J, Muller D, Harris P, Wattley L. *Nursing children: psychology, research and practice*, 3rd ed. Cheltenham: Nelson Thornes, 1999.

If you refer to the reference by Jones more than once during the essay, it will always be 1. For example:

> Two studies on children in hospital by Harris[11] and Jones[1] have looked at the need to prepare children prior to their admission . . . .

or

> Two studies on children in hospital[1,11] have looked at the need to prepare children prior to their admission . . . .

Cited works

The above examples show the uncomplicated use of the Vancouver system. There are, however, instances when it is not quite so simple. For example, if you have used the book by Taylor, Muller, Harris and Wattley, which refers to a study by Hawthorn, you should reference it as follows:

> A study by Hawthorn[5] looked at the nursing care of children in hospital.

The reference list would give the reference of the book by Taylor *et al* as:

5. Taylor J, Muller D, Harris P, Wattley L. *Nursing children: psychology, research and practice*, 3rd ed. Cheltenham: Nelson Thornes, 1999.

It would not in the above instance be appropriate to reference the Hawthorn study directly because you are discussing what Taylor *et al*. have written about Hawthorn's work, not your own interpretation of it.

(Where there are more than two authors, it is usual in the text to use the first author's name followed by *et al.*)

Edited works

Many books are written by a group of authors, who contribute individual chapters, with an overall editor. This can pose problems if you are referring to a chapter within an edited book. The usual format is to refer to the chapter author in the text but to refer to the book editor and title in the reference list. For example:

> Writing on the needs of the adolescent, Taylor and Barnes[6] discuss the need for health education material to be age appropriate.

The reference would be set out as follows:

6. Taylor J, Barnes K. Care of the adolescent. In: Barnes K, ed. *Paediatrics: a clinical guide for nurse practitioners*. Oxford: Elsevier Science, 2003: 190–199.

The Harvard style

The Harvard style again indicates the source of information within the text but, instead of using numbers, the author's surname and the year of publication are given and the full reference is included at the end of the work. For example:

> Children in hospital should spend time with their parents (Smith 1990). Hawthorn (1975) advocated this idea and it has since been reiterated by other researchers in this field (Rowe 1990, Wells 1987).

At the end of the work references are then organised into alphabetical order as follows:

Hawthorn, P. (1975) *Nurse, I Want My Mummy*. RCN, London.
Rowe, J. (1990) No place like home. *Nursing Times*, **89**(4): 14–15.
Smith, S. (1990) *Children in Hospital*. Hodder & Stoughton, London.
Wells, R. (1987) Staying in hospital. *Nursing*, **15**(6): 23–25.

Cited works

As with the Vancouver system, there are complications when you wish to mention an author whose work is referred to in a journal article or book but you do not have a copy of the original work. The work would be referred to as follows:

> A study by McDaniel and Wolf (in Grohar-Murray and DiCroce, 1997) examined the effects of transformational leadership on work satisfaction and retention . . . .

In the reference list you would refer only to the work of Grohar-Murray and DiCroce:

Grohar-Murray, M.A. and DiCroce, H.R. (1997) *Leadership and Management in Nursing*. Appleton & Lange, Stamford, CT.

Edited works

As with the Vancouver system, edited works can cause problems. If you were referring to a chapter written by an author in an edited work using the Harvard system, it would be as follows:

> Taylor and Barnes (2003) discuss the role of the nurse as a health educator with adolescents.

In the reference list it would be listed as follows:

Taylor, J. and Barnes, K. (2003) Care of the adolescent. In: Barnes, K. (ed) *Paediatrics: A clinical guide for nurse practitioners*. Elsevier Science, Oxford.

These two referencing styles are relatively simple and are usually used in a standardised way. It is, however, worthwhile checking with your lecturer if you have any problems.

The advantage of the Vancouver system is that you can put in many references at once without breaking up the flow of the text, while the Harvard system allows the knowledgeable reader (such as your tutor) to identify the sources you are using without constantly having to look up the reference list. It is also much easier to redraft your text if you don't have to renumber the references.

> ## Over to you
>
> Go to the library and see if you can find a journal that uses Vancouver referencing and one that uses Harvard. Make a note of the differences in style.

Electronic referencing

Increasingly, students are using the Internet and CD-ROM as sources when writing essays and producing other assignments. Similar principles apply as above depending on the referencing style. In the reference list at the end of the essay you should include the following:

For a CD-ROM reference

- Author(s)
- Title
- CD-ROM
- Journal Information
- Abstract/Index entry (with sufficient information to allow another person to access the reference).

For an Internet reference (include these if you can – it is not always possible)

- Author(s)
- Year
- Online
- Edition
- Place of publication
- Publisher
- Web address
- The date you accessed the source.

References and bibliographies

One final point. *References* are those works that are actually mentioned in your essay. A *bibliography* is a list of further material that has not been directly mentioned by you but has given you background information and may have influenced your work. A combined list may under certain circumstances be acceptable but it is always best to find out what is required before submitting the work.

~~Key points~~ **Top tips**

When referencing:

- If there are one or two authors only, both names should appear in the text and in the reference list.

- If there are more than two authors you can use the first author's name plus *et al.* in the text but in the reference list you should always write the names of all authors as they appear on the title page of a book or in the heading of a journal article.

- If you reference a book, you should always include the place of publication and the publisher in addition to the author(s), date of publication and title.

- If you reference a journal article, you should include the volume number and the part number (if there is one) of the issue from which the article came. It is not usually acceptable to write the date of the issue in a reference list. You should also include inclusive page numbers when you reference journal articles, as well as the author(s), year, the title of the article and the journal title.

- If you reference a book, you should underline the title of the book or place it in italics. If you reference a journal you should underline the journal title (e.g. *Physiotherapy*). You shouldn't underline/italicise chapter titles in edited works.

- Many books are reprinted either in their original form or as updated editions. If the book has been reprinted but not published as a subsequent edition, the first date of publication is the date you reference. However, if the book has appeared as a new edition (suggesting that the text has been updated and amended) you should reference the edition you have used. For example, *Study Skills for Nurses* in its first edition is simply referenced as Taylor (1992). It has been reprinted a number of times over the years without changes being made to it and it should still be referenced as Taylor (1992). However, if changes have been made to the text in 2003 and it appears as a second edition it will need to be referenced (in the Harvard system) as:

Taylor, J. (2003) *Study skills*, 2nd edn. Nelson Thornes, Cheltenham.

RRRRR*Rapid recap*

Check your progress so far by working through each of the following questions.

1. Identify two things important to the layout of an essay.
2. What factors should you consider when thinking about the style of your essay?
3. What are the essential differences between writing at levels 1, 2 and 3?
4. What is the main purpose of providing a reference?

If you have difficulty with any of the questions, read through the section again to refresh your understanding before moving on.

References

Buzan, T. (2000) *Use Your Head* (Millennium edition). BBC Books, London.

Eichler, M. (1988) *Non-sexist Research Methods: A practical guide*. Allen & Unwin. London.

Kirkman, J. (1992) *Good Style: Writing for Science and Technology*. E. & F.N. Spon, London.

QAA (2001) *The Framework for Qualifications of Higher Education in England, Wales and Northern Ireland*. QAA, Gloucester.

Further reading

Macdonald, J.W. (2000) *Report Writing*, 2nd edn. Croner, Kingston-upon-Thames, Surrey.

Walsh, M. and Wigens, L. (2003) *Introduction to Research*. Nelson Thornes, Cheltenham.

Projects, seminars and presentations

During your course you may be asked to present a seminar, make a presentation or submit a project for assessment. This chapter looks in detail at projects, seminars and presentations and gives practical information about each. The first thing to note is that in each case you should seek guidelines from the lecturer who sets the assignment so that you are aware of the criteria for assessment.

Projects

The term 'project' can take on many different meanings so if you are asked to undertake one you need to clarify exactly what is expected of you. A project usually takes the form of an extended essay with supporting diagrams and tables. These can be used to give visual impact to support written information and also as a way of presenting statistical information.

Students are usually given some choice about the exact topic for a project although some limitations may exist depending on whether it is part of the assessment for a single subject area or is part of a course. For example, as part of a sociology module you may be asked to undertake a project looking at an aspect of social class. Your exact choice of title may be left up to you. Alternatively, as part of a post-qualifying course you may be given a completely free choice about the topic area and will be able to choose a subject that is interesting and useful for you both personally and professionally.

If possible, you should ask for a tutorial so that you can check your plan and ensure that your proposed project is suitable. The lecturer may also be able to give you advice about where to find information. An example of a project plan is given in the case study on page 71.

One way of setting out your timescale is to use a **GANTT chart**.

A GANTT chart showing the stages for Clare's project is shown in Figure 7.1.

Keywords

GANTT chart
A visual way of demonstrating what tasks need to be done in a project and by when

Key points **Top tips**

Projects:

- Remember that you may be working on your chosen project topic for several months, so choose a topic that interests you
- Whether you have limited or free choice about a project title, you should always draw up a plan, which should include the following points:
  - The title
  - The aim(s) of the project
  - The themes you will be looking at
  - Supporting information, e.g. diagrams, graphs
  - Your time scale.

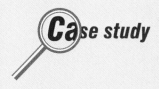
Case study

Clare's project

Clare is a nurse on a postqualifying child-care course and has been asked to undertake a project over a 6-month period, with a maximum word limit of 3000 words. She is given a completely free choice of topic and decides to look at HIV infection in children. She chooses this because it is a topic that she finds interesting, she feels she ought to know more about it and she is aware that there is sufficient published material for her to use. Her plan is as follows:

Project title: HIV infected children – the role of the nurse.

Project aim: The project will explore the needs of HIV-infected children and their families and will discuss the implications for the nurse in the clinical setting.

Themes:

1. *What the human immunodeficiency virus is.*

2. *The historical perspective.*

3. *How children become HIV-infected; vertical transmission, infection from blood, blood products and bone marrow, sexual transmission.*

4. *The natural history of HIV in children.*

5. *The needs of the child and family; physical needs, psychological needs, social needs.*

6. *The role of the nurse.*

Supporting information: Diagram of the virus; graphs illustrating statistical information about the virus; diagram of a child showing potential manifestations of AIDS; case history; nursing care plan showing physical precautions to prevent the spread of the virus in hospital.

Time scale:

Month 1 – literature search to be completed and requests sent.

Month 2 – all literature and other information gathered.

Month 3 – review literature and sort according to themes.

Month 4 – write first draft. Have tutorial.

Month 5 – final draft of main text to be completed.

Month 6 – supporting information completed.

Throughout the project preparation period, journals will be checked monthly for newly published relevant material.

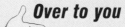

Over to you

Design a GANTT chart for your next assignment and try to stick to it.

Key points | **Top tips**

When undertaking a project:

- It should be logically set out with headings to break up the text.
- Diagrams and tables should be clearly labelled and should be situated with relevant text.
- Literature used should be clearly and accurately documented. A reference list and further reading section should be included at the end of the text.
- Any material included as appendices should be referred to within the text and included at the back of the project, after the further reading section.
- The project should be bound according to the guidelines, e.g. stapled, in a folder.
- Pages should be numbered.
- A title page should be included, giving the title of the project and your name, as well as other information requested in your guidelines, e.g. the date of submission, the course being followed.
- It is useful for the reader if you include a contents page listing the main headings and subheadings used in the project. You cannot complete this until you have written the project.

Task	Jan	Feb	March	Apr	May	Jun
Literature search to be completed and requests sent	▨					
All literature and other information gathered		▨				
Review literature and sort according to themes			▨			
Write first draft. Have tutorial				▨		
Final draft of main text to be completed					▨	
Supporting information completed						▨
Check journals monthly for newly published relevant material						

Figure 7.1 *GANTT chart showing a project schedule*

For further information about how to present both written and statistical material, see Chapter 6.

Seminars

A **seminar** can take the form of a brief formal presentation about a given topic followed by discussion, or can be totally participant-led. All those attending should be given the opportunity to put forward ideas, opinions, questions and solutions. It is advisable that all participants should come to the seminar with background knowledge and thoughts about the proposed topic.

The seminar organiser does, however, have additional responsibilities, which are outlined below. These guidelines should be used in addition to those issued by the subject teacher.

Preparing the environment

There are some aspects relating to the environment that you need to consider.

The seating arrangement is important and can encourage or inhibit group participation. If the chairs of participants are behind desks with the seminar organiser at the front, the impression will be of teacher and student rather than equal participants. Chairs placed in rows will often result in those at the back not being included in the discussion and participants will not be able to have eye contact with each other. The most satisfactory arrangement is circular or semicircular, which emphasises the equality of all those present. If a brief presentation is to be made, the speaker should be seated near the audiovisual equipment, e.g. overhead or data projector, video recorder. Other participants should be asked to move their chairs back for the presentation and close the circle during the following discussion.

Audiovisual equipment required should be checked before the seminar to ensure that it is in good working order. If a video is to be used it should be loaded into the recorder and the starting point should be found. Slides should be loaded and the focus checked.

Initiating discussion

If the organiser intends to make a presentation in order to trigger discussion, material should be prepared in advance and should be clear and relevant to the topic area. It is sometimes useful to highlight the anticipated discussion points using an **acetate** on an overhead projector at the start of the seminar. This gives some structure to the proceedings and can be useful if discussion relating to one topic area dries up. It is also useful for summing up and the organiser should ensure that an acetate pen is available so that unanticipated discussion topics can be added to the list.

Clarifying language and defining terms

The seminar organiser should ensure that a dictionary and other relevant literature is available so that issues can be clarified as they arise. It is useful for participants if the organiser provides a reference list of key texts so that they can follow up points after the seminar.

○━┳ *Keywords*

Acetate
The transparent 'paper' used to write on when using an overhead projector

Key points **Top tips**

When writing on acetate:

- Your writing should be larger than usual.
- Only include key points (not more than six or eight).
- Try not to write too close to the edge of the acetate.
- Use a piece of lined paper underneath the acetate so that your writing is straight.

Summarising seminar content

At the end of the seminar the organiser should sum up key points.

Follow up

Following the seminar the organiser should ensure that relevant information is circulated to participants. For example, if an issue was raised about which there was no information to hand, the organiser is responsible for finding the appropriate literature and circulating the reference to participants.

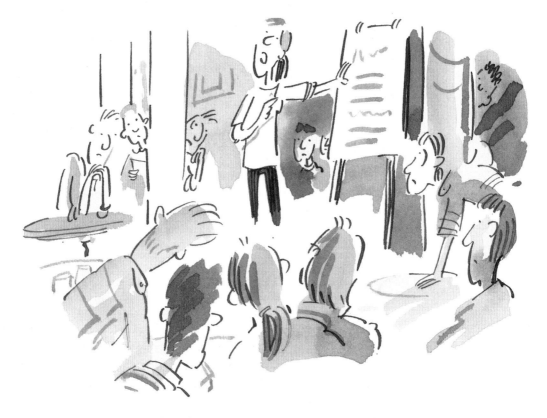

Don't forget to choose an appropriate room layout when leading a seminar

Presentations

During your course you may be required to make a presentation to peers. This may be an oral presentation, a poster presentation, a video or other form of work.

Oral presentation

If you are asked to make an oral presentation there are a number of essential things you need to find out:

- What is the topic you must present?
- How long have you got for the presentation?
- Are you expected to leave time for questions?
- How many people will be in the audience and who are they?
- What audiovisual aids will be available?

The next stage is to plan the main themes of the content. You might start by looking at the title of the presentation and underline the keywords. You then need to head to the library and search for information (see Chapter 3). How long you have for your presentation will determine how much depth you need to go in to. Don't swamp yourself with too much information if you only have a 10 minute slot.

Planning for the delivery of your presentation is vital. If you are going to cover three themes, draw up a plan of what information is going to be presented under which theme. Don't, however, turn your presentation into three disjointed sections – develop links between the themes as you identify them in your plan. You might say, for example;

> When I spoke about . . . a few moments ago I mentioned . . . .
> This is also significant to my second theme because . . .

or

> This links back to what I was discussing earlier and occurs in a similar way . . . .

After you have the main things that you are going to say, you need to practise vigorously. Some people are able to memorise speeches and can give presentations without the benefit of notes but most of us mortals have never mastered that art. I use a number of prompts depending on whether I am using audiovisual aids or not. If I am using acetates or a data projector, I have a large printed copy of each slide and I write prompts against each point on the slide. If I have to stand and give an oral presentation without aids, I feel that shuffling paper when all the audience has to look at is me is somewhat distracting, so I use prompt cards that I can glance at to remind me of what I need to say. Make sure that you number these (nervous presenters have been known to drop them) or do what I do and punch a hole in the top left hand corner and secure them with a Treasury tag. How much information you need to write down depends on you – if you are very familiar with the information you are going to present then just write down key words. Don't be tempted to stand and read – it means you do not interact with your audience, who will probably be asleep after 5 minutes.

Once you have chosen your preferred method of prompts, practise using them to make your presentation. Practise on your own in front of the mirror first and then subject friends and family to a run-through when you are fairly proficient. Ask them to be critically honest about any mannerisms you display and about things that you say that might have a double meaning or be confusing. Don't force your friends to listen hundreds of times or you will have a few less friends and fewer people to help you in the future! Time yourself to make sure you can present the information in the correct time.

When it comes time to make your presentation and you feel word-perfect, you are comfortable with your appearance and the stage is set, try to RELAX. Check audiovisual equipment in advance, make sure you have the right pair of glasses (if you need them) and read through your prompts. Wait until you are invited by the chairperson to take the stage and then remind yourself again to RELAX. The audience will feel your tension. Remember the pleasantries of thanking people for their time and interest, set out what you are intending to do, and then do it! A good tip is to focus on one or two people in the audience (preferably someone near the middle of the audience so that everyone feels included) and remember to smile. If you make a mistake, people will understand but be honest and don't try to bluff. My standard response if I make a mistake is to say something along the lines of 'what I should have said there is . . . . I'll make sure I get it right if you ask me again!'

A couple of final points. People like humour, but be careful. Don't attempt jokes that are likely to offend anyone in the audience (avoid sex, race and religion). And clear the decks when you have finished – remove your acetates, notes and any other debris so the next nervous speaker doesn't have to start his/her presentation by wading through your mess.

Key points **Top tips**

When making oral presentations:

- Check audiovisual aids in advance. Are they plugged in? In focus?
- Wait until the chairperson invites you to begin your presentation
- Try to relax!
- Thank people for attending and their interest in your presentation
- Outline what you are intending to do, what subjects you will cover, etc.
- Focus on a couple of people in the audience, preferably in the middle of the room
- Admit it if you make a mistake
- Be wary of using humour and avoid jokes based on sex, race and religion
- After your presentation, clear away your prompts, visual aids, etc. for the next speaker.

Poster presentations

A poster presentation is sometimes selected as a form of assessment for students, either on its own or supported by brief written information. You may be able to verbally explain your poster but this is not always the case. You need to ascertain whether you will be able to support your presentation before you decide what you are going to present. Clearly, if the poster has to stand on its own (without supplementary written or verbal information) it will have to be more self-explanatory. You also need to check clearly the guidelines for making the poster before you begin.

Don't be fooled into thinking that posters are judged on artistic flair and that if you are a good artist you can get away with little background work. Posters need to be accurate and informed and the *content* will be judged. The presentation is important, of course, but the information within the poster is more so.

The first stage of poster design is to do your background reading on the subject and decide on the key themes for your poster. Don't try to put too much on the poster – simple is good, so decide on what needs to go in. Have a go at sketching a few plans to illustrate ideas and ask other people for their thoughts too.

Once your ideas for your own poster presentation are starting to take shape, have a few 'dummy runs' with pieces of paper cut to the size (and shape) that you think your poster will eventually be. Don't forget that posters don't have to be oblong or square – you can come up with original shapes. Colour is also very important so think about whether there is an obvious colour scheme and, if there is, think about whether you want to go for the obvious. Unless you are trying to create something that looks like a children's toy box, try to avoid too many colours. Try different colour combinations on your practice sheets to look at different effects.

You might also decide that you want your poster to be interactive, for example, with flaps that observers have to lift to find answers. I have seen one poster with a buzzer fitted to a fairy light that was attached to a battery secured behind it! I designed a poster once to demonstrate the changes that occur in the fetal heart following birth with red, blue and purple stick-on plastic arteries. It took days to make but it was very effective. There really is no end to what you can do.

When you finally decide on all the attributes of your poster and have put together a final draft, ask a friend to look at it critically for you. Then put the finishing touches, think about paying to have it laminated (most stationers will provide such a service but it can be quite expensive) and make a protective cover for it. It really is heartbreaking if it gets ruined on the way to the presentation because it rained and the colours ran.

Key points **Top tips**

When doing a poster presentation:

- Is the poster going be displayed on its own, or are you providing supporting information?
- Get some ideas from posters and adverts around your neighbourhood
- Make up a few practice posters to see how it all fits together
- Think about the colours and shape you use – simple is often best
- Ask a friend to look at it critically for you
- Think about how to protect it – you don't want it ruined on the way to the presentation!

RRRRR*Rapid recap*

Check your progress so far by working through each of the following questions.

1. What is the purpose of a GANTT chart?

2. List the things that a seminar presenter should do.

3. Recap the development of a poster presentation from start to finish.

If you have difficulty with any of the questions, read through the section again to refresh your understanding before moving on.

Succeeding in practice

⚲ *Keywords*

Primary care
The first level of care, e.g. GP surgery

Secondary care
The second level of care, e.g. outpatient clinic or hospital ward

Tertiary care
The third more specialised level of care, e.g. rehabilitation settings

P ractice is an experience that most student health-care practitioners look forward to. It is, after all, what most people take a health-care course for. It is also a change of scenery, a chance to meet new people and most of all an opportunity to put some of the theory you have learned in lectures and seminars into practice and observe the reality of what health care is about. Even if you have already had experience of practice before, when undertaking a new course of study you will have new skills to try out and will see practice from a different perspective.

Your practice is likely to take place in a variety of different settings – primary, secondary and occasionally tertiary care areas.

In this chapter we will focus on the first two, as you are more likely to experience your earlier placements in these areas. A typical primary care setting would be a GP practice or health centre. A typical secondary care setting would be a stroke unit, acute ward or a fracture clinic, working alongside the first-contact practitioner.

It does not matter where you are in your training or where your placement is, all practice is worthwhile, all people you meet will have some influence on you and every opportunity should be seen as one to learn from. This includes the experiences that you feel are not important or not interesting. Most students enter training with some idea about where they would like to eventually work but it is useful to see all your other practice opportunities as experiences that will help you to become a 'rounded' professional. Remember that, in the real world of health care, patients move to and from primary, secondary and tertiary care and, while most professionals specialise in one particular setting, they need to be aware of other services and what patients will experience on their patient journey.

This chapter aims to help you to get the most out of your practice experiences whether in primary or secondary care settings and gives some useful hints about how to overcome some of the difficulties you might encounter.

> ## Over to you
>
> Before reading further, access the Department of Health website (www.doh.gov.uk) and find material on the 'Shifting the Balance of Power' development within the National Health Service.

Primary care

Practice placements in primary care provide an opportunity for you to get out and about. You may be attached to a rural practice, which will involve meeting and treating isolated groups of people. You may equally be attached to an urban one, where you meet people who live 30 seconds from the surgery. Primary care is not only about general practice. You may be attached to a particular health-care practitioner who is based in secondary care but who works in primary care, or you may find your placement is a community hospital, as these are increasingly being used for **intermediate care** within the health services. Some universities also place students in industry, schools, nurseries and call centres.

Wherever the practice, you need to be realistic about travelling and costs. You probably won't be allocated to your own practice where you are a registered patient and so it is realistic to expect to have to travel. Travel can be expensive and while you may be able to claim back travel costs you will most likely have to pay them yourself first. For some students this can amount to several hundreds of pounds. If you know you are going to have difficulty meeting these costs then make sure you talk to your tutors to see if they can help you. Universities don't want students to have to make choices about whether they can afford to eat or travel to placements. They want you to do both and they will only know if you are having problems if you tell them. A final point about travel is that, if you are using your own car for travel to placements, make sure you are insured for business use. Some universities will ask for a copy of your insurance policy but even if they don't you must be covered. This costs a few extra pounds on your premium.

The benefits of being on placement in primary care is that the working hours are unlikely to be 7am until 10pm and you will not usually be asked to work weekends, as you will in secondary care, although there are some exceptions to this. The beauty of primary care is that the practice staff team all know each other, are likely to have worked together for a while and have strong communication channels. As one of only a few students, they will get to know you (and your name), have a lot of time for you and plan your learning

Keywords

Intermediate care
Care provided (usually) by nurses either at the patient's home or in community care centres for patients who don't need high-dependency care in a hospital but still need some intervention

around you with the other team members rather than having to fit you in around other students' learning needs.

There are, of course, expectations that others will have of you. When you are introduced to people, try very hard to remember their names and roles, which can be a major problem for many people. However, people are flattered if you remember them from one meeting to another so it is an easy way of impressing people. Roy Sheppard, in a very useful book called *Meet, Greet and Prosper* (2002), provides some really useful hints for remembering names. His suggestions include the following.

- Really listen when someone tells you their name – most of us are nervous when meeting new people and this seems to adversely affect our memory.

- Imagine that you will be called upon to introduce the person to someone else within the next few minutes – try focusing on their first names at least.

- Ask the person to repeat their name if you didn't catch it first time round – if it is a difficult name ask them to spell it for you.

- Silently repeat the name to yourself. Some people find it useful to imagine a visual association with a name – this is easier with some names than others. It is also useful to link the name with the role, e.g. Peter Roper the Podiatrist, Debbie Andrews the Practice Manager. I find it useful particularly, if it is a difficult name, to find a word that the name rhymes with (a friend always used to introduce herself as 'Helene – rhymes with obscene!' – and no-one ever forgot).

> ### Over to you
>
> The next time you meet a group of new people, try some of the strategies for remembering people's names.

Primary care will put all your skills to use. You will be meeting and learning from medical practitioners, nurses, midwives and health visitors. A vast amount of experience and learning opportunities are available for you. This also applies to the patients you will be meeting, from the pregnant woman to the elderly gentleman with hypertension, from the teenager who wants contraception advice to the neonate with suspected meningitis. You will see and learn more than you could ever imagine.

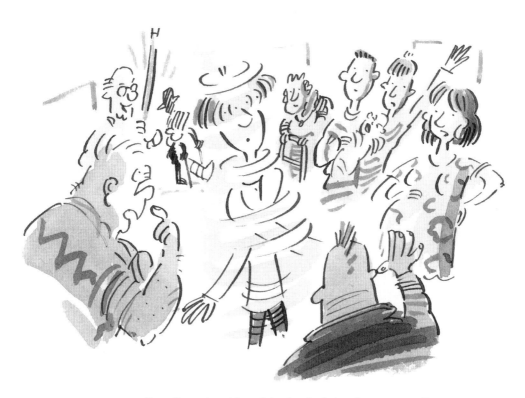

You will meet a wide variety of patients in primary care settings.

Primary care is likely to involve more observational work than within a hospital setting. You have the opportunity to observe people within their own environments and, while this can be shocking sometimes, it helps you to understand that the influence of the environment upon health is very important.

Over to you

List five ways in which an individual's environment could affect their health.

Another plus of primary care is that many practitioners who work in this setting will have taken on extended roles within their scope of practice and additional educational programmes to support their work. Make the most of learning from these individuals.

Over to you

You will probably already have been a consumer of primary care (as a patient at your GP surgery). Try to recall the services that general practice offers (or if you shortly have to visit the GP, make observations).

A placement in primary care is an experience that many people enjoy. Although not everyone will be suited to working in the community, you should try to get the most out of this area as throughout your career you will be constantly having to access primary care for your patients – for example, making referrals to the district nursing service or accessing GP surgeries for information on your patient.

Your time in primary care may be short and could be the only time in your working lifetime that you ever experience work within a community. You must remember that never again will you have such an amazing learning resource available to you. Primary care settings usually have the whole multidisciplinary team under one roof and you have personal access to all of them. Make sure you spend time with all the members of the team – individually they will have a great deal to teach you – and make sure that you learn about different approaches to work. For example, look at how the GPs communicate with and gain information from their patients in 10 minutes and then see how the nurse does this – learn from the different techniques you see.

Reflective activity

In your own life, have you been aware of health promotion and education activities, either at school, in the workplace or in your own GP surgery? Did it affect your lifestyle? If not, how might it have been carried out more effectively?

It will probably be the first time that you will have cared for people who are not necessarily acutely ill. Health promotion and health education make up a great part of the primary care team's role. The importance of this is that these practitioners have the time to do this and, more importantly, have knowledge of the person they are treating. They have a relationship with them and their families and know about their social, cultural and domestic lives. This is an observational dream – just watch the communication and interactions.

Keywords

Health needs assessment
An assessment of a community's health-care issues and its health services, from which a plan is formed of the priority areas needing improvement

Assessments in the community

One of the things you may be asked to produce as part of your community placement is a **health needs assessment** and community profile. Students are frequently asked to undertake this sort of assessment because it enables you to really appreciate the impact of an individual's living conditions upon their health. It also allows you to see how local health and social services are planned and prioritised to meet the needs of the local population.

> **Over to you**
>
> Look in the library and see if you can find a journal article that has undertaken a health needs assessment. Identify the steps that the authors took.

A health needs assessment is a means of identifying the priorities for health services within a population and then planning to address those needs in order to bring about improvements for the population as a whole. Health needs assessment is likely to take into account the views of consumers as well as professionals and will utilise a range of information. This will include audit data, information from the local authority about the age profile of the population, for example, and other numerical information such as mortality and morbidity. Each primary care area produces something called a Health Improvement and Modernisation Plan, which will help you to access some of the information you require.

The aims of the health needs assessment are therefore to:

- Include a range of key stakeholders and involve the local population/community
- Use information from a number of local agencies
- Be objective and systematic
- Make recommendations for change.

Figure 8.1 shows how the health needs assessment of the local community works.

Other documents that it may be useful for you to access within your primary care area are things like the Capacity Plan, the Local Delivery Plan and Workforce Development Plan. Most of these documents will be made readily available to you and if they are not offered, then ask!

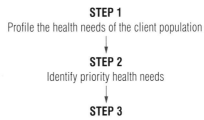

STEP 1
Profile the health needs of the client population

↓

STEP 2
Identify priority health needs

↓

STEP 3
Systematically assess each priority health need for change and agree action

Figure 8.1 *Health needs assessment of the local community.*

The health needs assessment will also help your understanding about the primary care area you are working within. It will provide you with:

- Insight into the health and social care experiences of the patients and clients you meet
- Insight into the strengths of the community and available resources
- Knowledge of local boundaries
- Insight into the impact of health policies
- Insight into the needs of carers
- Understanding of problems relating to access and equity
- Day-to-day contact with interested parties
- The ability to identify existing and emerging patterns of need
- The ability to provide **contemporaneous** data
- Evidence of effectiveness and cost effectiveness of local interventions.

Keywords

Contemporaneous
Existing in the same (or the present) time frame

Over to you

Think about how you would do a health needs assessment of your own locality. Remember, undertaking a health needs assessment is useful to you but will have been done before and most of the data will already exist in some form or another. Don't re-invent the wheel but find out what information exists, and ask for a copy. Some of the information will be easily accessible on websites, other information will be available only by seeking out the right people and asking them for it.

Key points Top tips

When on placement in primary care settings:

- Make the most of being one of only a few students on placement in the setting
- Don't forget that you'll be working with virtually the whole multidisciplinary team – use their many experiences and viewpoints to expand your own
- Enjoy meeting such a wide variety of patients and the diversity of health-care issues
- Make a note of the impact the environment can have on a person's health
- Consider what issues a health needs assessment of your placement locality might include

Secondary care

The majority of your practice will happen within a hospital with people who are acutely ill or have been so recently. Within this setting you will encounter nearly everybody you could think of, from the labouring mother to the terminally ill patient, from the refugee who doesn't speak English and can't understand you to the substance abuser who has taken an accidental overdose. The hospital placement will open your eyes to areas of people's lives you would not normally see.

Before your placement in a ward setting, make contact with the practitioner you have been allocated to. Turning up the afternoon before to collect your 'off duty' does not do you any favours. Unless you request a particular 'off duty', you will have been given a set of shift patterns. A ward area requires a set number of staff of the appropriate skill mix for each shift. However, within that framework there are now many opportunities for flexible working arrangements post-qualification. Try and work as many shifts with your assessor as possible. This is for your benefit – your assessor will not be able to assess your competence in relation to the learning outcomes regarding drug administration if s/he has not seen you assisting with a drug round or supervising a patient who is self-medicating.

It is also always useful if you know what the ward does.

Many wards make welcome packs for the students they have on their wards. These often include shift times, what the ward specialises in, what the student is expected to do and the ward philosophy. If your ward doesn't have one, often the hospital will have produced a student pack giving the same information but in more generalised terms.

The first days in an acute setting can be stressful, daunting, quite scary and exhausting. This does only last a few days. One of the biggest problems you will face is the large number of people – both staff and patients – with whom you will interact. Do not worry if you are unable to learn everyone's names and roles in the first few days. Concentrate instead on your assessor/supervisor/mentor and other students. You will also work with other members of the multidisciplinary team, such as the house officer from the medical ward.

It is worth trying to learn where things are stored and the usual routine and flow of the work pattern of the clinical area.

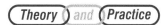

Theory *and* **Practice**

If you are allocated to a medical ward that specialises, for example, in respiratory conditions, why not read up on acute respiratory conditions such as asthma and chronic obstructive pulmonary disease? The staff in the area will appreciate the fact that you have taken an interest and are taking some time to learn about their speciality.

Theory *and* **Practice**

An acutely or critically ill set of patients may make the ward staff very busy, but despite this there is still a need for drugs to be administered on time to patients, hygiene needs to be met, etc.

No matter how busy a ward is, the overall routine for each shift will be roughly kept to. The quickest way to learn in this first week is to observe and spend time with your assessor and to assist with what is happening. Try not to jump in with two feet – take your time, as it will pay off.

Before and during the first week of your placement, your observations should allow you to think in more detail about what you want to learn from your placement. These learning objectives should be aimed at getting the most of your placement for your benefit. Things that should be considered include:

- Spending time with any specialist nurse
- Time in clinic to identify the pre-admission care of patients
- Following a patient (this is possibly more suited for surgical wards) throughout their hospital experience
- Attending and observing clinical investigations
- Spending time with the multidisciplinary team.

The wide array of learning opportunities will be facilitated by your assessor, who will identify what activities will be most beneficial at your particular stage of training. However, you should and must be able to justify why you are doing these things, as you must be able to justify all your actions while in practice. Throughout your initial health-care education you are given the opportunity to experience a wide range of clinical settings, from quite specialised areas such as Accident & Emergency and operating theatres to more general wards caring for patients with medical and surgical conditions. All the different areas in hospitals have their own unique learning opportunities and you are likely to prefer one speciality to another. Observe the role of the qualified health-care practitioner, as this will help you to conclude which area you would like to work in when qualified.

Your role as a practising student is fairly simple. You are there to learn. You should always be aware of your limitations and be willing and able to say when you cannot do something. Try and be aware of what is expected of you. This can be found in your learning objectives. Do not fall into the trap of saying yes to everything. If you have heard that someone else in your group has been giving intramuscular injections and you have not, do not panic – they have probably just been on a type of placement area that you will be in the future. Remember that you will do everything at some point. The golden rule is to see as many procedures as you need to before you feel confident enough to attempt one. For example, observe injection technique for as long as you feel it is necessary, then attempt to give

Key points **Top tips**

When on placement in secondary care settings:

● Don't try to remember everyone you meet – concentrate on your assessor, other students and a few key staff

● Make a note of your learning objectives for the placement

● Know your own limitations – don't be tempted to do what is beyond you

● Observe procedures until you feel confident enough to try them yourself

an injection (following guidance from your learning objectives, university and assessor).

Managing assignments, exams and your life while in practice

Everyone has their own way of managing their time and life and this usually works. Occasionally, people fall down when something unexpected happens in their life, but they cope, deal with it and move on, normally without too much damage being done. Don't be too hard on yourself as you begin your placements. Remember that, in practice, you are dealing with your life outside of work, your work as a practising student, assignment deadlines, and the other people's stresses, concerns, emotions and lives as well.

Rapid recap

Check your progress so far by working through each of the following questions.

1. What are some of the strategies for remembering people's names?

2. Give two examples of primary and secondary health-care settings.

3. What is a health needs assessment?

4. Make a list of those things that you ought to do before you start a placement in secondary care.

If you have difficulty with any of the questions, read through the section again to refresh your understanding before moving on.

Reference

Sheppard, R. (2002) *Meet, Greet and Prosper*. Centre Publishing, Clapton, Somerset.

9

Examination techniques

⚏ Keywords
....

Professional bodies
Organisations that regulate particular professions and the admission of candidates to the them

As health-care education has moved towards continuous assessment, the emphasis on a single final examination has been removed. This does not mean, however, that you will no longer have to pass examinations, rather that examinations will only be a part of the total summative assessment for the course. This chapter looks at the various formats of examinations and at how you can prepare yourself to be successful. You should, however, always check the format of examinations with your lecturer so that you are aware of what is expected of you.

Some **professional bodies** have rules about the inclusion of examinations in programmes as it remains the only simple way of ensuring that work produced is the student's own. Universities are, however, permitted some degree of flexibility in how they plan examinations. This flexibility may mean that you have advance notice of topics, or that you are allowed access to information during examinations. Summative examinations may well still include an unseen element so that, while you may be aware of the topic, you will not know the wording of the question. Some universities still have totally unseen examinations with no prior notification of topics. Many courses also include examinations in the form of OSCEs – objective structured clinical examinations to test clinical skills.

Some courses use new and innovative examinations involving technology, e.g. interactive computer assessment, video. Others may include face-to-face examinations with one or more examiner. These are sometimes mandatory (i.e. all students will have one) or selective (for students who are perhaps on the borderline of a particular grading band).

The preparation for different styles of examination will differ in some areas and the specific preparation is discussed in the following section.

Preparation for examinations

Unseen examinations

If your examination is totally unseen there are several factors you need to identify before commencing your revision programme:

- What format does the examination take (short answers, essays, etc.)?
- How long will you have for each question?
- Are there any revision sessions planned before the examination?

When you have clarified this information you can then plan out a revision programme so that your work is spread out evenly and you do not have to 'cram' at the last minute. When you devise your plan you should work out how many topics you wish to cover and the amount of time you have to work in. You should be able to work out how long you can spend on each topic. Preparing for essay questions is probably best tackled individually and it is useful to look through past papers or make up your own essay questions to identify the sorts of question that are likely to arise. Check your practice answers with your lecturer.

Mind mapping is a successful way of revising for answering essay questions under examination conditions and Buzan (2000) cites the extraordinary success of students who have accomplished mind mapping techniques. Mind mapping starts from a central theme, which branches out with related ideas. Ideas are logically followed through and, by using key 'recall' and 'creative' words or phrases, the map can be easily remembered.

Buzan defines a key 'recall' word or phrase as 'one which funnels itself into a wide range of special images and which, when it is triggered, funnels back on the same images'. A key 'creative' word is defined as 'one that is particularly evocative and image forming . . . but [does] not necessarily bring back a specific image' (Buzan 2000, p. 86).

Thus by using a combination of key recall and creative words within a map, you can remember the main points around which you can construct an essay. Examples of mind maps are given in Figures 9.1–9.3. Note that they include numbers to indicate the order of the themes for the essay. Figure 9.2 also includes pictures that enable you to visualise the themes for the essay.

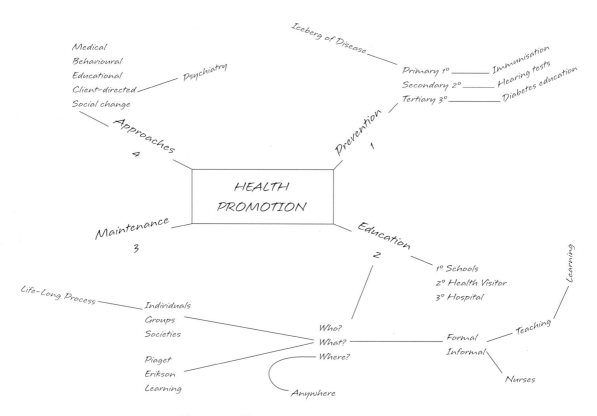

Figure 9.1 *Mind map – health promotion*

Top tips

Mind maps:

- Mind maps are a useful way of assessing yourself during your preparation period
- You can assess yourself in a wider range of material than if you spend time writing lengthy essays
- After you have designed your map, test yourself by reproducing it from memory and checking it against your master map.

As the examination draws nearer it is useful to write some timed essays. You can either start with a new topic and do a map plus an essay or you can take a map already constructed from your prior revision and write a timed essay from that. Remember that your map has a purpose and you should use it to prioritise points, structure paragraphs and stop yourself wandering away from the subject. It is important to do timed essays so that you can submit them for

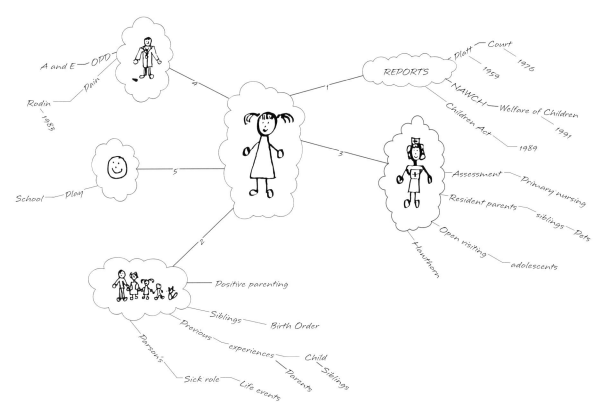

Figure 9.2 *Mind map – family-centred care*

marking and get feedback on your essay technique and content. If you cannot get a teacher to mark your essay, ask a colleague to look at it for you. If the feedback indicates that you have omitted a theme, add it to your map.

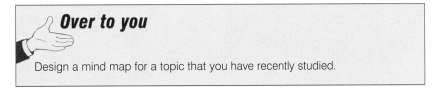

Over to you

Design a mind map for a topic that you have recently studied.

Planning for short-answer questions can be done individually in a similar way but on a smaller scale. It is also useful to join forces with colleagues and have non-competitive quizzes and joint brainstorming sessions. This is a pleasant and unstressful way of revising and will give you a break from individual work. It is also useful for identifying areas that several group members may find confusing and tutorial help on a group basis can then be sought.

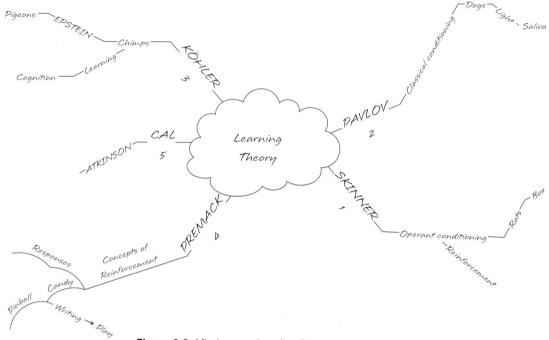

Figure 9.3 *Mind map – learning theory*

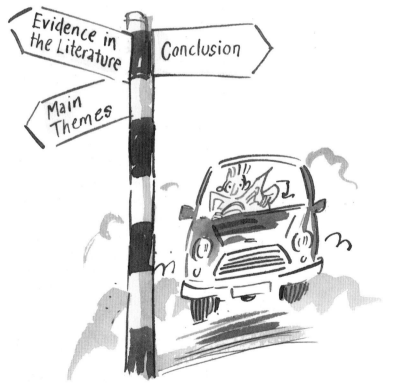

Mind maps are a good way of navigating your way through the themes of a subject

Seen topics – unseen questions

Seen topics should in theory narrow down the breadth of subject matter that you need to cover. However, giving seen topics usually means that you will be expected to produce a higher standard of work and show evidence of relevant reading. If you are given four topics and know you have to answer one, you should study one topic in depth but it is a good idea to have a 'reserve' topic in case the unseen question for your main topic is totally unrelated to what you have revised.

After you have decided on your main topic and your 'reserve', you need to collect your information. You may already have some information in notes and books and you should undertake a literature search (Chapter 3). This will enable you to show evidence of wide reading and you should try to remember author names. It is not usually necessary to remember direct quotations and full bibliographical details of sources. If you can remember the date of the work it is also helpful but not usually essential unless you are referring to a particular report or set of statistics (e.g. the OPCS infant mortality statistics for England and Wales in 1985, the Black Report of 1980, etc.). It is important to remember that lecturers can ask you, after the examination, to give the full information on a reference (e.g. the reference about child abuse by Smith).

Although the topic might be known, the exact wording of the question is not and you should therefore try and identify possible questions. The procedure for writing unseen questions then applies. This involves designing a map, writing and then submitting timed questions for marking. A useful way of remembering authors' names is to design your map with the names as your recall words (see page 94).

Accessing literature in the examination

Many universities allow students to access literature in summative examinations, and students are permitted to take a limited number of books and articles with them. Alternatively, universities may allow students to take a defined amount of notes into the examination, e.g. one side of A4 paper with notes. If you are allowed to use literature you should ensure that you are totally familiar with the material, and in the case of a book you should spend time before the examination using the index as a way of accessing information. There is a great variation in the style and detail of indexes and in an examination it is important that you can access information quickly and efficiently.

If you are permitted to take brief notes with you, mind maps are an invaluable source of information and they do not take up very much space. It is possible to recall far more information from a map than from written prose. It is also possible to do several mind maps on one piece of paper using different coloured pens – the maps can be written on top of each other and you will still be able to follow them. As with the other forms of examination, try to write some timed answers using your maps and submit them for marking before the examination.

The examination

Few people, regardless of their advance preparation, enter an examination room without feeling at least slightly apprehensive. The following section gives some advice about what to do when the dreaded time actually arrives.

Written examinations

Disciplining yourself to follow a few simple guidelines at the start of the examination can prevent apprehension turning into panic. Figure 9.4 shows how to undertake an examination in a systematic and calm way.

1. Turn over the paper and read the question – **twice.**
2. Draw appropriate maps learned during revision period.
3. **Re-read the question.**
4. Check information in the question, e.g. if the question gives a case history, note relevant points such as the age, marital status and social class of the patient.
5. Make further notes or add numbers to map to indicate the order of answer(s)
6. Write a note indicating when to finish writing each answer. Allow at least five minutes at the end for reading and correcting spelling and grammatical errors.

Figure 9.4 *The systematic way of taking an examination*

Writing your answers

While you are actually writing your answers you should constantly refer to your map so that you do not stray from the question. It is important that you cover a good breadth of material within your question but you should balance breadth with depth. Many universities award marks for the level of analysis demonstrated as well as for evident knowledge. If you are writing an essay answer, you should also remember to include an introduction and conclusion (see Chapter 6).

When you have completed your answer, or when you are within 5 minutes of the end of your allocated time limit, you should carefully read what you have written. Correct any obvious errors and then refer back to your map to ensure you have not forgotten any major points. Ensure that all your pages are numbered and that your name or examination number appears on each page.

Key points **Top tips**

When taking an examination:

- Read the question at least twice
- Draw mind maps if appropriate and number the topics in the order in which you will write them
- Make a note of any important information, such as patient details in a case history
- Write a note of the time you need to finish each answer
- Allow yourself 5 minutes at the end to read your work and correct any obvious grammatical errors

---

Objective structured clinical examinations

Objective structured clinical examinations (OSCEs) are designed to enable you to demonstrate the achievement of clinical skills in a simulated environment. The OSCE will usually take the form of clinical 'stations' through which you progress. Each station will present you with a different practical situation and will be designed to enable you to demonstrate skills in such areas as history-taking, physical assessment and examination, diagnosis and management of disease. At each station you may be required to interpret pathological, microbiological and biochemical information, etc.

Key points **Top tips**

When taking an examination:

- Don't forget that the OSCEs will usually require you to demonstrate 'caring' and communication skills as well as factual knowledge

---

Preparing for the OSCE is not unlike revising for a traditional examination but it is useful to be able to practice dextrous, communication and other skills under timed conditions. There are books that can help with this (see the Further Reading section at the end of this chapter) as well as computer packages.

⚷ Keywords

Viva voce
A face-to-face examination

Viva voce

A **viva voce** is required for certain qualifications (such as doctorates) but may also be used where a student is at a borderline of a grade. The viva is used to enable students to raise their grade (it rarely results in the opposite). For most the viva will be based on previously submitted work and the examiner or examiners will ask specific questions about it. Preparing for a viva is difficult, as you may be asked about any aspect of the work. The best advice is to be fully familiar with what you have submitted. This might sound fairly logical and obvious but it is amazing how much you can forget if the time between submission and the viva is lengthy.

When you enter the room where the viva is to be held take time to get settled and composed. Make sure you have with you a copy of your assignment, a piece of paper and a pen. When examiners are asking you questions, take note of them – particularly if the question is complex. In a state of nerves it is easy to forget what the start of the question was by the time the examiner has finished asking it! Don't be afraid to ask examiners to repeat questions or to rephrase a question. Better not to 'waffle on' about something you have not been asked about or understood! Remember to refer to your work and it is helpful to place self-adhesive notes to allow you to access sections of it quickly.

After the examination

Try to avoid talking about the examination with your fellow students (if you can), as this can cause unnecessary anxiety. Two students can take very different approaches to answering a question and still both pass. If you are genuinely concerned, ask for a tutorial and discuss your worries with your lecturer.

Key points **Top tips**

When taking a viva:

- Make sure you familiarise yourself with the assignment you have been asked to comment on
- On arriving, take your time to get settled and feel comfortable
- Ensure you have brought the assignment with you, along with a pen and paper
- Write down questions as examiners ask them, so that you don't forget what you're answering
- Don't be afraid to ask for a question to be repeated or rephrased
- Refer to your work throughout the viva – self-adhesive notes will save you trawling through your assignment to find the important sections

Key points **Top tips**

How to pass examinations:

- Carefully plan your programme of preparation.
- Seek tutorial help if you have any worries before the examination – most universities enable you to seek advice and most lecturers would rather see you before the examination to sort out your problems than afterwards when it is too late to help you
- Try to get a good night's sleep before the examination and have something to eat before you start – many examinations last for several hours and can be very tiring
- Ensure that you have a watch so that you can work out your timing for each part of the examination
- Make sure you have a couple of pens that you feel comfortable with and a supply of correction materials (if permitted)
- A few glucose sweets, a drink and a packet of tissues are also essential items – dehydration can affect concentration
- After the examination, remember that you cannot change what you have written so try not to worry about failing – wait for the results, which will tell you if you really have anything to worry about

RRRRRRapid recap

Check your progress so far by working through each of the following questions.

1. What is the difference between a recall and a creative word?

2. List the things you need to take to an examination with you.

3. What must you do when you get in the examination room before you start writing?

4. Give a brief description of an OSCE.

If you have difficulty with any of the questions, read through the section again to refresh your understanding before moving on.

Reference

Buzan, T. (2000) *Use Your Head* (Millennium edition*)*. BBC Books, London.

Further reading

Dornan, T, and O'Neill, P. (2000) *Core clinical skills for OSCEs in medicine*. Churchill Livingstone, Edinburgh.

Rowntree, D. (1998) *Learn How to Study*, 3rd edn. Time Warner, London.

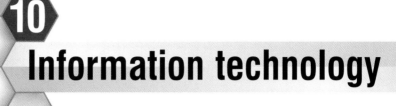

Information technology

10

Learning outcomes

By the end of this chapter you should be able to:

- Understand the basic components of a computer
- Appreciate the variety of packages and systems available
- Conduct searches on the Internet.

Information technology (IT) or, more recently, information communications technology (ICT) increasingly plays a significant part in our everyday lives and in particular within study skills.

This chapter looks at the use of ICT as an aid to study and does not go into the technical areas of computing. If you want to know more about bytes, ROM, RAM, CPUs, etc. you need to investigate the subject in its own right and this is best done outside of the confines of this book. Within this chapter we will look at the use of ICT within the following areas:

- **Computer hardware**: types of computer, operating systems, printers and peripherals
- **Computer software**: programmes that can be run on your computer – word processing, databases, etc.
- **Communications and imaging**: the Internet and the Web, digital photography and e-mail
- **Training**: different courses and training packages to allow you to get the best from your computer.

The aim of the chapter is to give you an understanding of the range and capabilities of the systems and software available to you.

Computer hardware

Computers come in all shapes and sizes – however in general terms there are two types: desktops and laptops. Both have their merits and you should consider these before making your purchase.

- The desktop:
    - Is generally more powerful
    - Has a larger VDU (visual display unit – screen size) capability
    - Has more memory and storage facilities (it can run more programmes and multitask)
    - Is cheaper than its laptop equivalent.

- The laptop:
    - Is portable and can be used almost anywhere (although battery life is generally limited to 3 hours)
    - Can undertake most of the applications of a desktop.

Both types are found with either of the two most common operating systems – PC (usually Microsoft Windows) or Apple Macintosh. The Macintosh operating system tends to be favoured for graphics applications; however PC is by far the more common.

Remember that these systems are not compatible and will not easily allow you to read work produced on the other system. In particular, PCs cannot read Macintosh disks. You should consider this when purchasing your new computer.

Computers store software programmes and any of the files that you produce on its hard drive. The storage capacities of these now run to tens of gigabytes (GB), which will far exceed the everyday requirements of most students. However the speed at which your computer processes information and its storage capability while doing this varies greatly with differing machines. The best advice is to buy the fastest processor (usually described as so many gigahertz (GHz)) and the largest RAM (memory) that you can afford. The World Wide Web, CDs and DVDs now contain excellent graphics and you may wish to download picture images from the 'web' or from a digital camera for inclusion within your documents, so make sure your computer has a good graphics card within its hardware specification.

You will also need other devices on your computer to transfer and store files that you produce. Originally these were 'floppy' disc drives but both CD and DVD drives are becoming more common as compact discs store considerably more information and are less easily damaged.

You may find that your college/university 'frowns' upon you bringing discs to use on their computers as many contain viruses – particularly if you use 'e-mail'. There are many free scanning programmes available and it is advisable to check your computer regularly by running one of these.

You will also need a modem to allow your computer to 'talk to' the Internet (many computers have modems built-in but they can be externally connected). Remember that to 'talk to' the Internet the computer needs a telephone line and unless you have a broadband connection that will allow talk on the telephone as well, no one will be able to use the telephone while you are 'surfing the Net'!

The other essential is a printer. Before purchasing, consider what materials you will want to produce. Printers vary in type

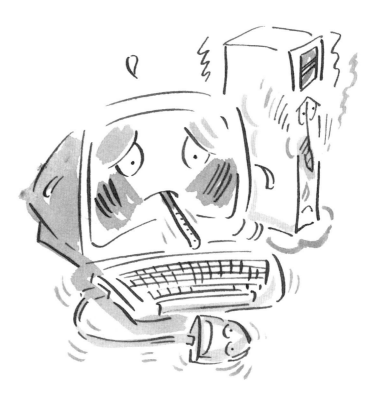

Don't forget to regularly virus-check your computer.

and specification, from simple ink-jet printers to sophisticated laser models that produce stunning hard copy graphics. Some printers can also act as a fax and photocopier. It is fair to say that you get what you pay for but, before buying what appears to be a bargain, check the price of the replacement ink/toner cartridges – your 'bargain' may in the long term prove to be very expensive!

Key points **Top tips**

Buying hardware:

- Before you walk into a computer shop, decide what tasks you want the machine to be able to do
- Does your computer need to be portable (you may want to able to take it with you to lectures) or can you leave it in a permanent place?
- Find out what free scanning programmes exist to prevent viruses from infecting your files
- Before buying a printer, check how expensive the replacement print cartridges for it are

Computer software

A computer's software contains the programmes that run on your computer. Typical packages include Microsoft Works or Microsoft Office. These packages include word processing software, which allows you to write your essays, spreadsheet software, which will allow you to do mathematical calculations and to display these as graphs and pie charts, database software that will allow you to build and interrogate your own information storage systems, and e-mail software through which you can send and receive electronic mail and other documents once your computer is linked into the Internet. Most computers have one of these (or similar) preloaded.

Other software that may also be pre-installed on your computer includes Internet Explorer, which, once linked through an internet service provider (ISP), such as AOL, will allow you to 'surf the Net' for information. The ISP usually offers an e-mail hosting service and will allocate e-mail addresses (e.g. superstudent@aol.com) for your use so that people can contact you. If you are studying at university or college, many will allow you to have an e-mail address on the college site (e.g. superstudent@college.ac.uk). You should contact the college ICT section to find out more.

Key points | **Top tips**

Computer software:

- Look at the programme software that comes with your computer. Is it adequate? Will it do the jobs that you want? It is cheaper to have software installed at the time of purchase than installed at a later date.

Communications and imaging

Although computers originally started out as simple 'number crunchers' and then developed further into word processors, recent years have seen them evolve into sophisticated communication devices. The growth of the Internet and the World Wide Web (www) has opened huge areas of information to the world at large. You can now find information on nearly any subject that you care to name through entering a query through one of the many search engines on the Web.

Search engines may well bring a response of thousands of 'hits' (sites that have information that relates to your query). From these you should be able to find the information that you require, on any

> ## Over to you
>
> Using a search engine (e.g. www.google.com), type in your particular health-care profession. Note the diversity of the sites that are found.

subject. However, a word of caution here – the web has no 'police' to enforce the accuracy or content of any sites. You will find information from the Department of Health (www.doh.gov.uk), the NHS (www.nhs.gov.uk) or other world organisation or agency but you may also find misleading or offensive material on some sites.

Key points **Top tips**

Searching on the Internet:

- When using search engines, be as specific as you can. If you simply type 'doh', hoping to find the Department of Health, you can be directed to over 20,000 sites dedicated to The Simpsons!

You will also find it useful to become familiar with *Boolean* searching. Boolean searching was named after the man who developed the principles on which the system is based, George Boole. Virtually all search engines recognise Boolean terms (O'Dochartaigh 2002). Boolean searching is based on the use of words that we use in everyday language: and, or, and not, not, near and *.

Key points **Top tips**

Using Boolean terms to search online

- If you want to search for documents that contain two words you use *and* e.g. children *and* audit.
- If you want to search for documents that contain either word you use *or* e.g. children *or* audit (don't try this as you will end up with thousands of hits!).
- If you want to search documents for a specific word and not another you use either *not* or *and not* (some search engines respond to one and not the other) e.g. viruses *not (and not)* bacteria.
- The Boolean term *near* is used to search for documents containing two key words but only if they appear within a few words of each other e.g. children *near* audit.
- Finally, * is used to search for documents containing words beginning with a particular stem e.g. audit* will include auditor, auditing and so on.

Key points **Top tips**

Using the Internet:

- If you want to use the Internet, make sure your computer has a modem.
- If you are going to use the Internet a lot, remember it is probably better to subscribe to an ISP that makes an inclusive monthly charge rather than one that charges for telephone line usage by the minute.
- Remember if you are 'on-line', people cannot use that telephone line. It may be worthwhile to have a dedicated Internet line or subscribe to a broadband service.

Training

This chapter has briefly looked at the types of computer (hardware) and what might help you in your study, the programmes (software) that you need to have on your computer to help you produce assignments and the information that is available to you to complete research for your assignments.

As with everything, you can only get the best from your machine if you are taught to use it properly. There are hundreds of IT and ICT courses available, from entry level (e.g. Computers for the Terrified) through to professional qualificatory awards. These can be studied at many locations near you (such as libraries or schools) or you may well find that your own college or university runs a course that will suit your needs. Alternatively your local bookshop or library will have some very useful user-friendly books on IT and you can teach yourself through these. Finally you can also develop your IT skills through one of the many government-sponsored schemes, such as the BBC's 'On-line' or UfI's 'Learn Direct', that you can access, through the Internet, on your own computer.

Over to you

Identify the areas within ICT where you feel your skills are weakest. Word processing? Spreadsheets? Using e-mail?
Go to your nearest college and find out about available training courses – better still, look it up on the Internet! As a guide, all schools and academic institutions have website addresses ending in.ac.uk (www.nameofcollege.ac.uk).

Key points **Top tips**

IT training:

● To get the best from your computer, you need to be 'IT literate'. If you do not feel competent or even confident, take lessons – self-study or evening classes.

● Remember – your computer may seem clever but it is not as clever as you! It can only do what you tell it to do, so if you don't know – find out!

Refle **Reflective activity**

Think about the course you are doing and identify what you actually need a computer to be able to do. Will you, for example, need complex graphic packages?

RRRRR Rapid recap

Check your progress so far by working through each of the following questions.

1. Identify the Boolean search terms you can use.

2. What are the advantages and disadvantages of buying a laptop computer as opposed to a desktop computer?

If you have difficulty with any of the questions, read through the section again to refresh your understanding before moving on.

Reference

O'Dochartaigh, N. (2002) *The Internet Research Handbook: A practical guide for students and researchers in the social sciences*. Sage, London.

Copyright

During your health-care course, it is important that ideas, thoughts and information are exchanged and shared with colleagues. However, the Copyright, Designs and Patents Act 1988 should be adhered to when sharing material that is copyright protected. The Act outlines when copies can be legitimately made and when you could be breaking the law. Parts of the Act are outlined below and a reading list is provided so that you can explore this subject in more depth if you wish.

What material does the Copyright Act protect?

- **Typographical arrangements of published editions**: this refers to the whole or any part of published literary, dramatic or musical works, including books, journals, poems, essays, songs, etc.
- **Original literary, dramatic, musical and artistic works**: this includes graphic works, photographs, maps, paintings, drawings and diagrams
- **Films, sound recordings, broadcasts or cable programmes**
- The Computer Programmes Regulations 1992 extended the copyright on literary works to include **computer programmes**

Who owns copyright?

The owner of copyright is usually the original author, artist, photographer, etc., except where the work was produced as part of someone's duties as an employee, in which case copyright belongs to the employer (subject to any agreement to the contrary).

The owner of the copyright of published editions is usually the publisher. This principle does not, however, apply to Crown or governmental publications. In these cases you are advised to seek clarification from the Stationery Office website (www.hmso.gov.uk) as to what you can copy and for which publications you would need a licence.

In the case of a broadcast, the person making the broadcast usually owns the copyright, and in the case of a cable programme, it is usually the person or people providing the programme service in which the cable programme is included (for example, UK Gold, E4).

Copyright can, however, be bought, sold or given away.

How long does copyright last?

This depends on which Copyright Act was in force when the work was published (pre-1957, 1957–1988, post-1989) and if the work was published when the author was living or dead. The following gives some indication of how long copyright may exist in some instances. However, check before you copy.

- Literary, dramatic, musical and artistic works are protected for 70 years from the end of the calendar year in which the author died. If the author was not still alive when the work was published for the first time, the work is in copyright for at least 70 years from that first publication date.

- Sound recordings are protected for 50 years from the end of the calendar year in which they were made or from the end of the calendar year in which they were released.

- Broadcasts are protected for 50 years from the end of the calendar year in which the broadcast was made or from the end of the calendar year in which it was first transmitted. Copyright on repeated broadcasts expires at the same time as that of the original broadcast.

- Published editions are protected for 25 years from the end of the calendar year in which the first publication of the edition was released.

- Crown copyright material published prior to 1989 is protected for 50 years after first publication. After May 1989, it is protected for 125 years from when it is made or, if commercially published in the first 75 of these years, for 50 years from the year of first publication.

It is not safe to make assumptions about copyright expiry – check with the copyright holder or the Copyright Licensing Agency before you copy.

What are you allowed to copy?

- You can make single copies of copyright material for private study or research provided that not more than a 'reasonable part' is copied. The Library Association interprets this as: 'One chapter or extract from books, pamphlets and reports amounting to no more than 5% of the whole work. Up to 10% of a British Standard, or two pages if the standard is short.'

- You can make a single copy of a periodical article but not more than one article from the same issue of a periodical. Most libraries ask you to complete a declaration form before you are supplied with a copy or allowed to make a copy.

- Permission is not needed to make hand-written or typewritten copies of text or illustrations for research or private study. It is also permissible to copy material on to a blackboard. It is generally accepted that it is permissible to make one overhead transparency or slide of copyright material for the purpose of teaching. However, the Copyright Act does not cover this medium.

- You may make copies of work that does not indicate who the copyright owner is as long as you have made reasonable attempts to trace the owner. Again, this should be for the purposes of research or private study.

- You may copy work that is not protected by copyright (usually because a number of years have passed and work is no longer protected – or occasionally you will find material that states it is copyright free).

- You may be able to copy some material if your establishment has a licensing scheme. You need to check the terms of the licence before you copy. If your establishment has a scheme but the work you wish to copy is not covered by it, special conditions apply, which you need to abide by.

- Educational establishments are allowed to take off-air recordings if the programme forms a part of the curriculum. Recordings cannot be taken of programmes that are covered by a licence, unless the establishment is itself licensed to do so.

- You may rewrite (but not photocopy) the abstracts of scientific or technical subjects that appear in periodicals.

Infringement of copyright

The copying of work is an act restricted by the Copyright Acts. This refers to:

- Reproducing in any material form, literary, dramatic, musical or artistic work.
- Copying in relation to a film, television or cable programme, including making photographs from them.
- Copying in relation to typographical arrangements of published editions.
- The making of an adaptation of work. This includes adaptations in recorded or written form.

Obtaining permission to copy works

How do you get permission to make copies that are not for private study or research?

The usual practice is to write to the copyright owner asking for permission to copy. You should include exact details of which part of the work you wish to copy, how many copies you wish to take and the purpose of taking the copies. It is usual to give assurances that the author will be acknowledged in your work. You must then wait until you have written, signed permission from the copyright owner before copies are taken. It is sensible to keep the original permission reply and, if payment is requested, you should ask for and keep a receipt of payments made.

Key points Top tips

- Copyright is designed to protect the livelihood of the creators and producers of literary, musical, dramatic and artistic work
- Infringing copyright is a breach of the law

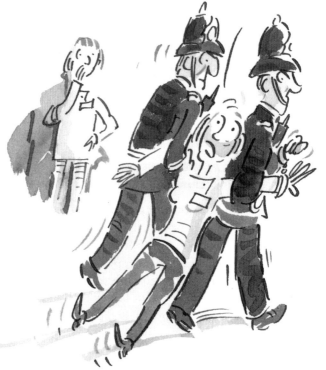

Check before you copy.

Top tips

Copyright:

- Always 'Think Copyright' before you copy anything – if something is covered by the Copyright Act, adhere to the law
- The restrictions on the copying and use of videos and published works are usually clearly stated at the beginning of the video, book or journal
- If you wish to ask permission to use material covered by copyright, allow an appropriate amount of time for permission to be granted – for example, if copyright belongs to a publisher in the UK allow 2 months and allow even longer for obtaining permission from other countries
- If you have any doubts about copying all or part of a published work, ask the librarian – libraries are issued with guidelines relating to the Copyright Act

RRRRRRapid recap

Check your progress so far by working through each of the following questions.

1. What comes under the copyright laws?
2. Where will you find the copyright restriction in a book?
3. How do you go about gaining permission to copy an item covered by the copyright laws?
4. What are the restrictions on copying for personal use?
5. Are computer programmes covered by copyright law?

If you have difficulty with any of the questions, read through the section again to refresh your understanding before moving on.

Further reading

Copyright, Designs and Patents Act 1988. HMSO, London.

Crabb, G. (1990) *Copyright Clearance – A Practical Guide*, 3rd edn. National Council for Educational Technology, London.

12

Essential skills for employment

Learning outcomes

By the end of this chapter you should be able to:

- Understand the aim of key skills and what they cover
- Compile a CV
- Prepare effectively for interviews
- Survive the interview process!

This final chapter aims to help you to enhance your chances of being employed at the end of your training – it may also provide some useful tips for getting a summer job on the way. The chapter starts by looking at key skills – essential employability skills for the future. It then looks at how to put together a *curriculum vitae* (CV) that will convince potential employers that you have these essential skills and encourage them to invite you for interview. The chapter concludes with some tips for succeeding at interview.

Key skills

There is increasing concern that programmes of education prepare students well within a defined subject area but do not produce employees who are able to function fully within the workforce. The Department for Education and Employment (2000) identified that the possession of a degree is not an indicator of competence for certain careers and that if graduates are to make an effective transition into the labour market they need to ensure that they develop their personal and employability skills. The NHS Plan (Department of Health 2000) suggests that much more needs to be done to ensure that educational programmes within the health sector produce practitioners who are both fit for practice and fit for purpose. This includes making sure that health-care students emerge from their educational experiences with employability skills to enable them to function fully and competently within the work place. In essence, students graduating from health programmes are no different from other graduates and steps need to be taken to integrate employability skills within health-care curricula.

Key skills of employability

The Dearing Report (1997) stated the belief that there are four skills that are key to whatever graduates intend to do in later life. These are communication skills, numeracy, the use of information technology and learning how to learn. The report suggested that these skills are not just relevant in employment but also throughout life.

The Department of Education and Employment (1998) defines key skills as the essential employability skills that people need to enable them to be effective members of a flexible, adaptable and competent workforce. Key skills are the generic, transferable skills that the government and much of industry consider to be essential for successful lifelong learning and for a flexible workforce (QCA 1998). The Qualifications and Curriculum Authority identifies six key skills, building on and expanding those skills identified within the Dearing Report (1997). These are:

- Communication
- Application of number
- Information technology
- Problem solving
- Working with others
- Improving own learning and performance.

There are five cumulative levels of keys skills identified ranging from Level 1 to Level 5. Table 12.1 defines the expectations for these levels.

○━☌ *Keywords*

Panacea
A universal remedy or cure-all

It is not suggested that the attainment of these skills will be the **panacea** for the overall problem. However, their attainment at the appropriate level will at least ensure that the government, the employer and the educational establishment can have confidence that you are competent in certain areas that supplement your specific academic knowledge. In addition, you will be able to approach potential employers with evidence that you have achieved a set of skills that will facilitate your induction to the world of work.

Table 12.1 QCA key skills levels	
Levels 1 & 2	Help to develop basic skills and increase confidence in applying skills to routine situations.
Level 3	Able to respond to more complex activities. Needs explicit reasoning ability and making decisions about own learning and organisation.
Level 4	Autonomy and responsibility for managing activities. Develop strategies for monitoring own progress, presenting outcomes and evaluating own performance.
Level 5	Demonstrating an integrated approach in applying all key skills. Managing dynamically complex work. Mostly self-directed.

The integration of key skills in health-care curricula

Key skills were introduced in many schools and further education colleges in September 2000, with the introduction of 'Curriculum 2000', although the uptake was not universal. In universities the introduction of key skills is less formalised and is working to a longer timescale. However, the Quality Assurance Agency framework on higher education qualifications (FHEQ; QAA 2001) is expected to become a formal code of practice, which means that universities will be expected to adhere to it. The current FHEQ states that courses within higher education should include 'qualities and transferable skills necessary for employment'. You can therefore expect to receive tuition in key skills development sooner or later.

Try not to think as key skills as yet another thing to learn – the whole purpose of key skills is that they will mostly be things that you will gain as a byproduct of your other learning. The advantages of them is that they can give employers confidence of the competence of potential employees in certain key employability skills. They also provide a springboard for lifelong learning and enhance the subject specific skills that students learn during their educational programmes. As a health-care student, skills such as communication, information technology and numeracy are essential if you are to be able to function effectively within the health services.

Over to you

Create your own self assessment tool. This is a way of assessing your own strengths and weaknesses. Using the six key skills areas as a guide, make a list of:
- Your current strengths
- Areas for improvement
- Actions you could take to increase your skills
- How increased skills will support your future studies and/or employment

Writing a CV

A CV is a tool to enable you to give a potential employer a sound understanding of your previous achievements and experiences. You should tailor your CV to the post you are applying for to ensure that you highlight your particular strengths that relate to the particular post. Remember that employers may receive many, many CVs and yours needs to stand out! The points in the Top Tips box aim to give you that edge to at least help you to get short-listed.

Key points **Top tips**

CVs

- Print your CV on high-quality paper and, when you send it off, keep a copy for yourself

- Keep the layout simple and consistent – it should look pleasing to the eye and should comprise a logical outline of your experiences so far

- Be honest – if you lie on your CV, you will probably be found out

- When you have finished writing your CV, check it for mistakes and get someone else to check it for you

- At the end, put the date on which you updated it (i.e. 'last updated 01/10/03')

- Keep your CV concise – busy managers do not want to wade through 20 pages

Essential and optional components of a CV

What to include on your CV really depends on you and whether you see a particular aspect of your experience as a strength or otherwise. The list below is not exhaustive and you will see that some items are considered optional. If your CV is going to support an application form, as is usually the case, delete or shorten any information that is duplicated. The headings will help you with the structure.

Personal details

Include here:

- Name
- Home address
- Telephone number(s) and e-mail address(es) – state which are home and which are work/daytime/evening
- Nationality (optional)
- Date of Birth (optional)
- Marital status (optional)
- Sickness record (optional) – if you do include a sickness record restrict it to the last 2 years and state the total number of days over how many occasions (e.g. 4 days in total taken on two occasions).

Educational qualifications

It is usual here to include the names and addresses of educational establishments attended, the dates of attendance, the examinations taken (including those you failed), the results (including grades) and the dates of the awarded results.

List these in order with senior school first, followed by further and higher level qualifications. If you are currently studying, follow the guidelines above but put the date you started followed by '– (current studies)'

Professional qualifications

Similar principles apply to the above. If you have a professional registration, include the professional body you are registered with, the Personal Identification Number, and the date of expiry.

Further training

You may wish to include other study and training that you have undertaken which has not led to a qualification, such as in-house development opportunities or training undertaken as part of voluntary work.

Employment history

Try to keep this brief but informative. When you have worked for the NHS for 25 years the Saturday job that you had in Marks and Spencer when you were 16 is not really important!

Put your current employer (if you have one) first, followed by your previous employers from the most recent back, giving inclusive dates of employment, your post, a *very* brief list of responsibilities, and the reason(s) why you left (e.g. 'promotion', 'moved area', 'to undertake course'). Most employers are only interested in the past 10 years.

Remember to explain any gaps in your employment history (e.g. '6 months unemployed due to travelling abroad for gap year'). Include at the end of this section any voluntary work that is relevant to your application.

Publications and research

If these are substantial then have two separate sections. If not leave them as one and if you have no experience then leave the section out.

If you do list publications and/or research then do so in logical order. Publications should be properly referenced. If you have been involved in research, indicate whether the research was funded or not and, if it was funded, by whom. If you were the lead researcher, indicate this. If research was undertaken as part of a course, then indicate this too.

Memberships, external committees

If you are a member of an organisation that relates to the post, or you have experience of working for an outside organisation, put this on your CV. For example, if you are a member of a committee or national working party, put the name of the committee, the date that you were engaged and your role.

Hobbies, interests, etc.

These are optional but if you do have an interesting hobby that might be relevant to the post you are applying for then include it. You don't want to make this section too exhaustive. Employers want you to sell to them the fact that you can do the job, not that your job supports a hobby – no matter how interesting!

Brief resumé of current responsibilities

This section is optional but in my experience useful. In particular, it can be adapted, depending on the job, to emphasise strengths in relation to the person specification/job description. Restrict it to one page and keep it concise.

> ## Over to you
>
> Compile your own CV and save it as a computer file so that it can be easily updated.

Preparing for an interview

Interviews are always stressful – don't let anyone tell you otherwise. You have a limited time to convince a group of strangers that you are better than lots of other people who are probably equally well qualified to do the job.

Preparing for an interview can be divided into five parts:

- What to wear
- Background swotting
- Last minute preparation
- Conducting yourself in the interview
- After the interview.

What to wear

As someone who regularly interviews people I know that this is a very important area. First impressions of a person are of their smartness (or lack of it). The job you are being interviewed for should influence your dress. This is generally much easier for men than for women – but not always!

The rules are common sense but it is worth noting them here. Try to go for 'smart' if you are applying for a professional position. If you are asked (as is sometimes the case) to attend an informal interview first you should still go for smart. – informal does not mean you can turn up in your jeans. Even if you only have one smart outfit and it means wearing it twice it doesn't matter. Try to wear a different shirt/blouse, tie/scarf to give a different appearance to the outfit. Get your clothes ready the day before so that you don't have to search through the ironing basket on the morning of the interview to find that lucky shirt.

Key points | **Top tips**

What to wear:

● Go for smart and simple: you don't want to distract the interview panel by your appearance – you want to sell them the idea that you have ability and experience

Background swotting

Most interviews will explore how the candidate matches the job description or person specification and you should be fully conversant with these and how you meet them. If you have completed an application form make sure you keep a copy and also take a copy of your CV. Match up areas that you feel you meet the job description and refer to those areas if asked. It is a good idea to write down examples, as interviewers are looking for evidence that you really do have experience. For example, if part of the job description is about managing conflict, you should have identified a recent example of how you did handle conflict and what the outcome was.

You should also read carefully any background information sent to you by the organisation and, if this is limited, see if they have a website. Read all the information carefully and refer to it in your answers. As you are swotting, write down anything that you are not clear about and when you have finished reading, form these into two or three short questions.

If you are asked to bring certificates, your passport or any other documents, make sure you have them ready to take with you in advance.

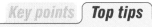

Background swotting:

● Take a copy of the application form and your CV along to the interview

● Make a note of where your experience and proven abilities match the job description and take this along

● Find out background information about the organisation and look at their website if they have one

Last minute preparation

Last minute preparation includes making sure you arrive in plenty of time so that you can have a drink, visit the toilet and read through any notes you have made. Try to be calm and be pleasant to the other candidates if you are asked to wait with them. Try to avoid discussing your previous experiences or why you are the better person for the job – and don't listen when others do this to you. The other candidates are not the interview panel but can make you feel totally inadequate before you even meet them!

Key points | Top tips

Last minute preparation:

● Arrive in plenty of time to find where you need to go, visit the toilet, etc.

● Try to avoid discussing previous experience with any other candidates who might also be waiting – it's likely to make you more nervous

Conducting yourself in the interview

At the beginning of this section I mentioned that interviews are stressful, so you need to try and manage your stress. Remember that all the candidates will be nervous so you are all starting off from the same base. The formal interview starts from the minute you enter the interview room, so walk into the room with confidence. If it seems appropriate, shake hands as you are introduced to the panel but if this is clearly not expected then don't. Smile at people as you are introduced.

Some interviewers still set the interview environment up like an interrogation and there is unfortunately little you can realistically do about this. Sit down when you are invited to and make yourself comfortable, being aware of your body language. Look people in the eye when they ask you a question and try to keep your body posture as relaxed as possible.

Answering questions is never easy under interview conditions and it is worth getting a friend to practise a few questions in advance and give you honest feedback about, for example, how many times you say 'um', how you wring your hands when answering, eye contact, and so on. Interviewers should ask you clear questions, which are not ambiguous. If you don't understand or you lose your drift, ask the interviewer to repeat the question. Interviews are contrary to every other aspect of life when you are taught to think carefully before you speak. You don't have the luxury of spending half-an-hour thinking about your answer in the interview. You have very little time but this doesn't mean you can't think.

Your answers to questions should be to the point and you should refer to your direct experience and the literature that the organisation has sent you, or that you have seen on the website. Don't wander off the point – if they don't ask you a question that you think they should have, you may have the opportunity to add this vital piece of information at the end – you can try to phrase it as a question such as: 'I have a great deal of experience in _____, which you mention in the job description. I was wondering how these particular skills would be utilised in practice?'

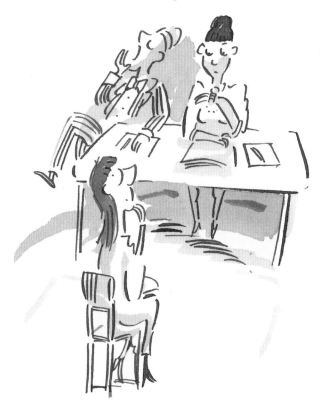

Take your time when answering questions, but not too much!

Key points **Top tips**

In the interview:

- Ask a friend or colleague to practise asking you 'interview' questions and to provide you with constructive feedback
- Smile at the interview panel as you are introduced and shake hands if appropriate
- Try to make yourself comfortable, with a relaxed posture.
- When answering a question, try to maintain eye contact with whoever asked it
- Give yourself time to think before answering a question, but not too much time!

After the interview

If you are offered the job, even if you know you want it, be sure to ask for a reasonable period of time to consider your response. Do you *really* want this job? Do you have any other interviews for jobs that you think you will like more?

If you are unsuccessful then you will usually be offered feedback. If you are told you haven't been successful, more or less straight away ask if you may seek feedback in a few days so that you have time to reflect on how you felt at the interview. When you seek feedback ask for specific information about why you were unsuccessful otherwise it will not help you when you prepare for the next interview. Write down the feedback and ask for clarification if you don't understand a particular point.

One final point – if you really liked the organisation and felt the interview procedure was good, and you think that you might apply for a job there in future, then a brief letter telling the organisation how much you valued the literature they sent or the way the interview day was structured will be appreciated and, who knows, may make a difference next time.

Key points **Top tips**

After the interview:

● If you are offered a job after interview, give yourself time to think before you accept or decline

● If you are not offered a job after interview, ask if they can provide you with feedback on your performance

● Write this feedback down – it may help you prepare for another interview

● If you were unsuccessful but particularly enjoyed the interview format, or tasks involved, there's no harm in writing to the organisation and saying as much.

RRRRRRapid recap

Check your progress so far by working through each of the following questions.

1. What is the purpose of key skills?

2. List the 6 key skill areas.

3. When writing a CV what should you include?

4. What advice might you give a friend about preparing for an interview?

If you have difficulty with any of the questions, read through the section again to refresh your understanding before moving on.

References

Department of Education and Employment (2000) *Skills and Enterprise Briefing*. DfEE, London.

Department of Health (2000) *The NHS Plan*. DoH, London.

Qualifications and Curriculum Authority (1998) www.qca.org.uk/nq/ks

Qualifications and Curriculum Authority (2000) *Guidance on the Higher Level Key Skills Unit*. QCA, London.

Qualifications and Curriculum Authority (2001) www.qca.org.uk/nq/ks

UKCC (1999) *Fitness for Practice*. UKCC, London.

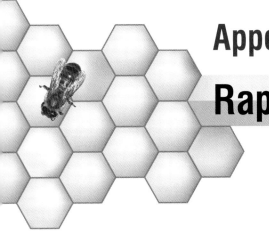

Appendix

Rapid Recap – answers

Chapter 1

1. **Make of list of things you should do to make sure you are comfortable in your study environment.**
   - Ensure you're not hungry or thirsty.
   - Ensure you have a comfortable chair.
   - Ensure the temperature is suitable for you to work in.
   - Ensure you have adequate lighting.
   - Ensure you have some privacy.

2. **Identify three things that you should consider when working in a group with other students.**
   - Choose a suitable venue.
   - Decide who is completing which bits of the work and by when.
   - Ensure that the team edits the work as a whole, to avoid inconsistency of style and duplication. Evaluate each other's performance within the team.

3. **Identify the seven sections of Maslow's hierarchy of needs.**
   - Self-actualisation needs
   - Aesthetic needs
   - Cognitive needs
   - Self-esteem needs
   - Belongingness and love needs
   - Safety/security needs
   - Physiological needs

4. **What is the difference between formative and summative assessment?**

   Formative assessment provides feedback on progress and development and does not count towards formal assessment of a course.

Summative assessment provides a measure of performance (either achievement or failure) and is related to the outcomes of a course.

Chapter 2

1. **What are the grants available to ensure that no student is excluded from higher education?**

   Grants for childcare, books and travel.

2. **What are the four different rates for the NHS Hardship Grants Scheme?**
   - A standard rate for non-mature students without dependants living outside London
   - A rate for mature students without dependants living outside London
   - A rate for non-mature students without dependants living in London
   - A rate for mature students without dependants living in London.

3. **What does NUS stand for?**

   NUS stands for National Union of Students.

Chapter 3

1. **List the points to consider before you start a search for information.**

   Clearly define the subject, decide upon the searching strategy, choose which libraries and information services are most appropriate and check if they are available, decide which sources of information are most suitable for the project.

2. **What benefits might LIS offer you?**

   LIS facilities provide access to a wide range of sources and resources. They are also run by staff qualified to help in finding specific material.

3. **What is a gateway or portal?**

   A gateway or portal is a website dedicated to a specific subject area to provide access to a number of websites on the topic.

Chapter 4

1. **What does SQ3R stand for?**

   Survey – Question – Read – Recall – Review

2. **What are the main aims of each (SQRRR)?**

   Survey: To take in headings, diagrams, tables and summarised sections.

   Question: To reflect on how the text contributes to knowledge already learned and decide on the important points to look for and what needs to be re-read.

   Read: To read the text more slowly but only the sections that are necessary to the work in hand. To look up words that aren't understood. To write definitions down so that they are not forgotten.

   Recall: To put the text into context of what is being studied. To summarise in brief note form the main points highlighted in the text and decide if there are areas still not understood.

   Review: To go quickly through the process of survey, questions, read and recall a second time – preferably after a break.

3. **What are the three most common ways of taking notes during lectures?**

   Summary notes, framework notes and pattern notes.

4. **What must you always do as soon as possible after a lecture?**

   (Not 'go to the pub'!) Read through notes, even type them up. This will help reinforce the information.

Chapter 5

1. **List six things to look for in a literature review.**

   Is the literature relevant to the study?

   How old is the literature? If it is old, does it matter?

   Does the researcher use literature from one country or from many countries? Does it matter?

   Is the literature described or does the researcher attempt to review each piece of literature and discuss its strengths and weaknesses in relation to the other literature reviewed?

   Does the researcher discuss the implications of the literature?

   Are the sources of the literature used clearly documented?

2. **What are the two major** *approaches* **to research?**

   Quantitative and qualitative.

3. **What is the purpose of undertaking a pilot study?**

   It acts as a trial run to the main research study, on a smaller scale.

4. **List four questions you might ask yourself about your overall impressions of a research study.**

   Was the study readable and interesting?

   Did it really achieve its purpose?

   Did it include any irrelevant material?

   Does it contribute to existing knowledge?

Chapter 6

1. **Identify two things important to the layout of an essay.**

   Any two of:

   Does the essay have to be typed or can you write it out? If typed, are there any stipulations about line spacing, e.g. double spacing?

   Can you write on both sides of the paper?

   What referencing style should you use?

   What information should you include on the title page, e.g. name or examination number, date, institution?

   Do you need to leave margins on one or both sides of the pages?

   Are there any other guidelines?

2. **What factors should you consider when thinking about the style of your essay?**

   Can you write in the first person?

   Avoid sexist language

   Write at an appropriate academic level

3. **What are the essential differences between writing at levels 1, 2 and 3?**

   Level 1 involves writing descriptively

   Level 2 involves writing analytically

   Level 3 involves writing a greater depth of analysis, i.e. critical analysis

4. What is the main purpose of providing a reference?

References provide the means for the reader of your work to go to the original work and read it for themselves to see how it supports your argument.

Chapter 7

1. What is the purpose of a GANTT chart?

A GANTT chart allows you to visually plan a project, showing what you have to achieve and by when.

2. List the things that a seminar presenter should do.

A seminar organiser should prepare the environment, initiate the discussion, ensure that a dictionary and other literature are present in case needed, sum up key points at the end of the seminar, follow up any issues arising from the seminar discussion.

3. Recap the development of a poster presentation from start to finish.

a.   Ascertain whether you will be able to support your presentation with documentation.

b.   Check any guidelines set for making the poster.

c.   Do some background reading on the subject and decide on the key themes.

d.   Try sketching a few plans to illustrate ideas and ask other people for their thoughts too.

e.   Have a few 'dummy runs' with pieces of paper cut to the size (and shape) of your final poster.

f.   Think of colour schemes.

g.   Will the poster be interactive?

h.   Put together a final draft and ask a friend to critically look at it for you.

i.   Add the finishing touches, possibly have it laminated and make a protective cover for it.

Chapter 8

1. What are some of the strategies for remembering people's names?

Imagine that you will be called upon to introduce the person to someone else within the next few minutes.

Ask the person to repeat their name if you didn't catch it first time round – if it is a difficult name ask them to spell it for you.

Silently repeat their name to yourself.

Link the name with the person's role.

Find a word that the name rhymes with.

2. Give two examples of primary and secondary health-care settings.

Primary care: for example, GP practice, health centre, walk-in centre

Secondary care: for example, critical care unit, stroke unit, surgical ward

3. What is a health needs assessment?

An assessment of a community's health-care issues and its health services. From this a plan is formed of the priority areas needing improvement.

4. Make a list of those things that you ought to do before you start a placement in secondary care.

Make contact with the placement setting well in advance of your arrival date.

Alert your assessor to any major events you already have planned that may affect your shifts.

Read up on the area of health-care the placement is concerned with.

Ask if the ward (or hospital) has a welcome pack for placement students.

Chapter 9

1. What is the difference between a recall and a creative word?

A recall word is one which at a certain time makes you think of a certain image and, when that word is triggered at a later date, the original image is recalled. A creative word is one which at a certain time makes you think of definite images but, when that word is triggered at a later date, you do not think of the original images.

2. List the things you need to take to an examination with you.

Pens, a watch, a drink, tissues, sweets.

3. What must you do when you get in the examination room before you start writing?

Read the question at least twice, draw a mind map, note any important information in case histories, etc., note the time at which you need to finish each question.

4. **Give a brief description of an OSCE.**

OSCEs are Objective Structured Clinical Examinations, which are practical examinations to test clinical skills.

Chapter 10

1. **Identify the Boolean search terms you can use.**

The Boolean search terms are 'and', 'or', 'and not', 'not', 'near' and '*'.

2. **What are the advantages and disadvantages of buying a laptop computer as opposed to a desktop computer?**

A desktop is generally more powerful, has a larger VDU capability, has more memory and storage facilities and is cheaper. A laptop is portable and can be used almost anywhere and can undertake most of the applications of a desktop.

Chapter 11

1. **What comes under the copyright laws?**

Published literary, dramatic or musical works, including books, journals, poems, essays, computer programmes, songs, etc.

Original literary, dramatic, musical and artistic works, including graphic works, photographs, maps, paintings, drawings and diagrams.

Films, sound recordings, broadcasts or cable programmes.

2. **Where will you find the copyright restriction in a book?**

This should appear on the imprint page at the beginning of the book (where details of the publisher and year of publication are given).

3. **How do you go about gaining permission to copy an item covered by the copyright laws?**

Write to the copyright owner asking permission to copy. Include exact details of which part of the work you wish to copy, how many copies you wish to take and the purpose of taking the copies. You must then wait until you have written, signed permission from the copyright owner before copies are taken. Keep the original permission reply and, if payment is requested, you should ask for and keep a receipt of payments made.

4. **What are the restrictions on copying for personal use?**

You should not copy more than 5% of the total of a published literary work. You may copy a whole periodical article, but not normally more than one article from each issue of a periodical.

5. **Are computer programmes covered by copyright law?**

Yes, since 1992.

Chapter 12

1. **What is the purpose of key skills?**

Key skills are the essential, transferable, employability skills that people need to enable them to be effective members of a flexible, adaptable and competent workforce.

2. **List the six key skill areas.**

The six key skills are communication, application of number, information technology, problem solving, working with others, improving own learning and performance.

3. **When writing a CV what should you include?**

The components to choose from for a CV are: personal details, educational qualifications, professional qualifications, further training, employment history, publications and research, memberships of external committees, hobbies, brief resumé of current responsibilities.

4. **What advice might you give a friend about preparing for an interview?**

Advise them to look smart, to do some background swotting on the job and organisation and to arrive in plenty of time.

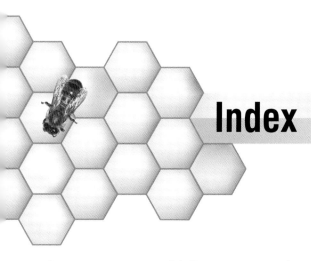

Index